SHORTNESS OF BREATH

A Guide to Better Living and Breathing

SHORTNESS OF BREATH

A Guide to Better Living and Breathing

ANDREW L. RIES, MD, MPH
KENNETH M. MOSER, MD
PATRICIA J. BULLOCK, RRT, RCP
TRINA M. LIMBERG, BS, RRT, RRP
ROSEANN MYERS, RN, BSN
DAWN E. SASSI-DAMBRON, RN, BSN
JAMIE B. SHELDON, PT

Division of Pulmonary and Critical Care Medicine
University of California–San Diego
School of Medicine

FIFTH EDITION

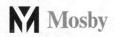 Mosby

St. Louis Baltimore Boston
Carlsbad Chicago Naples New York Philadelphia Portland
London Madrid Mexico City Singapore Sydney Tokyo Toronto Wiesbaden

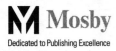

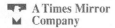

Vice President and Publisher: Don Ladig
Editor: James F. Shanahan
Developmental Editor: Anne J. Gleason
Project Manager: Patricia Tannian
Senior Production Editor: Ann E. Rogers
Book Design Manager: Gail Morey Hudson
Cover Designer: Teresa Breckwoldt
Manufacturing Manager: Dave Graybill

FIFTH EDITION

Copyright © 1996 by Mosby–Year Book, Inc.

Previous editions copyrighted 1975, 1980, 1983, and 1991

NOTE TO THE READER
A number of medications, exercises, and other forms of medical treatment are reviewed in this book. While the descriptions are as accurate as possible, they should not be taken as direct instruction or recommendation for any individual patient. The contents of this book are informational only. Any specific medication or exercise should be prescribed by a physician and initiated under appropriate medical guidance.

Printed in the United States of America.
Composition by The Clarinda Company.
Printing/binding by Malloy Lithographing, Inc.

Mosby–Year Book, Inc.
11830 Westline Industrial Drive
St. Louis, MO 63146

Library of Congress Cataloging in Publication Data

Shortness of breath: a guide to better living and breathing/Andrew
    L. Ries . . . [et al.].—5th ed.
        p.   cm.
    Includes index.
    ISBN 0-8151-7339-3
    1. Lungs—Diseases, Obstructive—Popular works.   I. Ries, Andrew L.
    RC776.03S53   1996
    616.2′4—dc20
                                                                    96-24648
                                                                    CIP

95 96 97 98 99 / 9 8 7 6 5 4 3 2 1

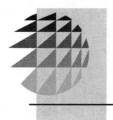

Preface

Any book with multiple authors of different backgrounds must have an interesting story behind it, and this one does. The story began more than 30 years ago, when we established one of the first Respiratory Intensive Care Units in the United States. Trying to save the lives of patients who had developed severe, life-threatening breathing problems was a rewarding and exciting venture. Yet we soon recognized that many admissions to this Unit, and to the Hospital, could have been avoided if the patients had, long before, better understood the causes of breathing problems and how to deal with them. We decided that educating patients was a vital and missing link in the health care system. Individuals with breathing problems were, almost exclusively, *passive observers* of their own health care. But we became convinced that, with proper education, people could and should become *active participants* in their own health care.

But how could laypeople acquire such education? Certainly not through medical textbooks, which were too technical and detailed. Nor through the standard media, which dealt only sporadically with breathing problems and rarely presented practical or scientifically sound information. Nor from most "health books," which usually presented a point of view rather than a body of facts. And not from busy physicians or other health professionals who, however well motivated, rarely had time to educate their patients. Furthermore, many individuals with breathing problems did not know when or whether to enter the "health care system" and, therefore, often entered it at a late stage with advanced problems.

So we concluded that such an educational effort could be provided most effectively by a team of health professionals that included individuals with a wide range of professional skills and knowledge: pulmonary physicians, pulmonary nursing specialists, respiratory therapists, chest physical therapists, cardiopulmonary technologists, psychiatrists, social workers, nutritionists, occupational therapists, and hospital administrators. This team would develop a course devoted to the education of patients with breathing problems, emphasizing the most common cause of this symptom: chronic obstructive pulmonary disease (COPD), but not neglecting those with other forms of chronic obstructive lung disease.

At that time, such ideas and approaches were controversial. Some felt that an educated patient might be more of a threat than a help to the health care system; others felt that people would not be interested in such self-education. Still others believed that such an effort would intrude on doctor-patient relationships. Despite such reservations, the effort was undertaken.

The multidisciplinary team was developed and together designed a course for people with shortness of breath and other breathing problems. The first individuals came, learned, and benefited. The process was refined, changed, and repeated, and a gratifying dividend appeared. As the years and courses passed, many physicians and other health professionals visited our program to learn the course elements so that they could begin similar efforts at their offices, clinics, and hospitals.

But an increasing source of frustration to us was that our efforts were still reaching a relatively small audience. Our program was consistently backlogged, and we could reach only a modest percentage of the interested individuals in our immediate geographic area; extension of our program to other areas was not feasible. This book was a logical means for extending our educational efforts to the larger audience that we could never reach in person.

So that is the story behind the first edition of this book, which appeared in 1975. Five years later, in 1980, the second edition of this book was published; in 1983, the third; in 1991, the fourth; and now, this fifth edition. With each edition, we have asked those individuals who have used this manual to help us make it more valuable to them. And we have listened closely to their suggestions this time as well. In addition, there have been medical advances in our understanding of the multiple lung diseases that can cause symptoms, as well as gains in treatment. One among many such advances has been the expanded availability and feasibility at our institution and others of lung transplantation for many patients with advanced breathing problems. And it has been found that participation in a rehabilitation program is a key element in the preparation of such patients for surgery—and in their postoperative maintenance.

So, over the years, this book—like all aspects of medical care—has changed. One thing, however, has not changed; indeed, it has become stronger. That thing is our belief that individuals with breathing problems can become active members of the treatment team, accepting (and enjoying) the fact that they can and must play a central role in their own care. That is still the theme of this book. In fact, since 1975, that theme has become a national one in the area of health care: the individual's *active participation* in maintaining and improving his or her own health.

We hope that all of our colleagues in medicine will continue to find this book useful and that patients with breathing problems will learn from its pages how to live better and more functional lives.

Of course, despite the multiple authorship, many others have contributed greatly, directly or indirectly, to this book. We owe special debts of gratitude to Steve Pileggi and Nancy Dimsdale, whose illustrations have contributed so much to our programs and to this book. In particular, we would like to thank the former staff members of the UCSD Pulmonary Rehabilitation Program who, over the years, have contributed to the development of the Program and as authors and contributors to previous editions of this book: Carol Archibald, R.N.; Deon Dunn, R.N.; Marion Modrak, R.N.; Patsy Hansen, R.N.; Alice Beamon, R.T.; Birgitta Ellis, P.T.; Donna Whelan, R.T.; Martin Davis, R.T.; and Lynn Johnson, R.N. Several psychiatrists and psychologists have devoted themselves to the mental health of our patients (and ourselves): these include Stephen Groban, M.D.; Alan Abrams, M.D.; and Sharon Grodner, Ph.D. Of the many allied health professionals who have shared their knowledge, this experience, and themselves, we would particularly like to thank dieticians Joyce Knott and Kelly Mosier, who have taught our patients and us so much about nutrition; pharmacists Richard Levy, Raffi Simonian, Ken Schell, and Joanne Goralka for straightening us all out about the proper use of medications; Jane Villareal, a social worker whose caring and understanding were exemplary; and a succession of pulmonary trainees and students at UCSD who have been our teachers as well as our students. For the publication of this book, we owe much to Vannessa Kennedy and Maureen Faraguna, who have borne the administrative burdens of translating our ideas into readable copy. Finally, most of all, we owe thanks to our many patients who have continued to return to us far more than we have given to them.

Andrew L. Ries, M.D., M.P.H.
Kenneth M. Moser, M.D.

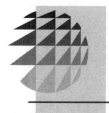

Contents in Brief

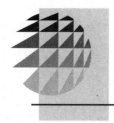

Contents

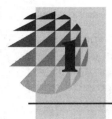

What Are Shortness of Breath and Other Breathing Problems All About?

Most of us take breathing for granted. Like the beating of the heart, breathing just happens automatically. When we exercise, we know our breathing quickens and deepens, just as our pulse rate increases. But again, we don't have to think about these things. We decide what we want to do and somehow the lungs and heart follow along.

The fancy medical word for feeling short of breath is *dyspnea* (pronounced disp'-nee-ah). Dyspnea is a difficult symptom for people to deal with because it is a feeling, or a sensation. Only the individual knows that he or she is experiencing shortness of breath. The physician also has trouble evaluating dyspnea. Often it cannot be detected on physical examination. There is no specific test for it. Therefore, the individual must report dyspnea to the physician. In many ways, dyspnea is like pain—a symptom that only the patient feels and can describe. Pain and dyspnea are invisible to others.

Like pain, shortness of breath is experienced differently by different people. Some individuals have a very high threshold for pain, some a very low one. It is the same with dyspnea. Some people who appear to others to be short of breath do not themselves feel dyspneic. Other individuals feel quite short of breath when they appear to be breathing normally. Just why this is cannot be fully explained. There are probably multiple reasons.

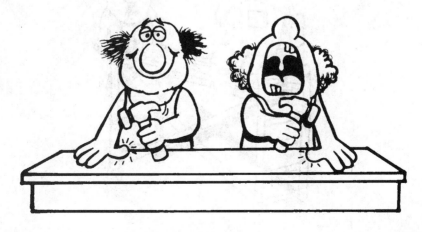

WHEN IS SHORTNESS OF BREATH ABNORMAL?

So shortness of breath is a tricky symptom. To compound the problem, everyone feels short of breath sometimes. Even the well-conditioned athlete with excellent lung and heart function experiences dyspnea. So how do you know when shortness of breath is abnormal? When is it a possible signal of disease? When should you have it checked out by a doctor?

Here are some simple tests to apply:

1. Are you more short of breath doing certain things than other people your own age are? It is obviously not abnormal when a 60-year-old man or woman feels short of breath while playing tennis with a 20-year-old son or daughter. It is not abnormal to feel short of breath if you lead a quite sedentary life and suddenly try to run a mile. But it is abnormal if you feel short of breath walking up an incline or up stairs when people of your own age (co-workers, friends, or spouse) do not. Comparison with peers is a key test.

2. Are you short of breath doing things that a few months or a year ago you could do easily without this feeling? Do you now avoid the stairs at work or home because of shortness of breath? In answering these questions, you are comparing you with yourself. The questions should be answered honestly. Denying such changes won't make them go away.

3. Have you experienced a sudden change? Suddenly feeling short of breath while resting or being active is almost always abnormal. A rapid change like this merits prompt medical attention.

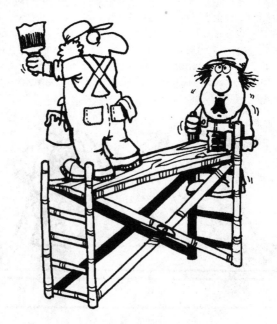

Asking these questions usually distinguishes normal from abnormal shortness of breath. Sometimes, though, the individual either does not ask these questions or denies that the answers are "yes." Or, unconsciously, you may cut back on what you are doing to avoid shortness of breath. In such situations, other people may have to call the problem to your attention. They notice that you are breathing hard during a walk at a pace that is leisurely for them. Spouses are often the first to notice such things. If friends or spouses pose these questions to you, take them seriously rather than explaining them away (which is easy to do). You may have a "high threshold" for dyspnea, but if you are changing your behavior to avoid shortness of breath, others may be more aware of it than you are. Or maybe you *are* aware, but you don't want to admit it as long as you believe that no one else notices.

CHECK IT OUT

However shortness of breath is called to your attention, it is better to take it seriously than to push it out of your mind. Taking it seriously means seeing a physician. The doctor can then check out whether the shortness of breath is normal or abnormal for you. As with most symptoms, delay in finding out about dyspnea is not wise. If there is something wrong, valuable time may be lost—time during which the chance for effective treatment may pass. If there is *not* something wrong, if you or others around you just have a "low threshold," then finding that out will relieve your mind—and theirs. Remember: "when in doubt, check it out."

WHAT CAUSES SHORTNESS OF BREATH?

If shortness of breath is a signal of disease, what are the possible problems involved? Well, there are a lot of possibilities—just as there are a lot of causes of pain. For example, anemia can make people short of breath, and anemia has multiple causes. Being overweight can cause dyspnea, as can certain glandular problems, such as an overactive or underactive thyroid gland. Heart diseases of various types are a frequent cause of shortness of breath—without chest pains or any other symptoms. But the most common reason for shortness of breath is lung disease.

All of the causes of shortness of breath can usually be sorted out by having a physician obtain a careful history, do a complete physical examination, and perform certain simple laboratory tests: a blood cell count, a chest x-ray examination, and an electrocardiogram. Sometimes more extensive tests will be needed to find out whether anything is really wrong and, if so, what it is. But the doctor also should take your symptoms seriously, not dismiss them with a statement that you are "getting older" or

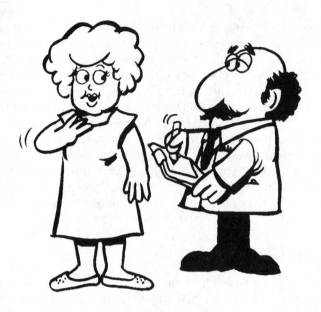

are "out of shape." The history and physical examination should be carefully done, and at least the three tests mentioned should be performed.

WHAT KINDS OF LUNG DISEASE ARE THERE?

If this sequence has been followed, and if the reason for your shortness of breath turns out to be the most common one—lung disease—you will want to know what kinds of lung diseases there are and what must be done to find out which kind you have.

There are many diseases that can affect the lungs and lead to shortness of breath. Most of them, particularly the ones with long and complex names, are rare. But despite the many possibilities, lung diseases can be grouped into three main categories: restrictive diseases that reduce the volume of the lungs, diseases that injure and/or block the blood vessels of the lungs, and obstructive diseases that make it difficult to expel air from the lungs (slow down exhalation).

The restrictive diseases cause shortness of breath by either scarring the lungs or filling their air spaces. Usually these diseases are slow and progressive—and so is the shortness of breath they produce. Sometimes the cause for this chronic irritation and scarring of the lungs is known: exposure to asbestos, beryllium, or other injurious fumes or particles or an allergic reaction to certain inhaled materials such as cotton dust or pigeon droppings. Such inhalation exposure most often occurs at work but may occur at home. Many of the restrictive diseases are of unknown cause. These are grouped under the term *idiopathic*—a terrific medical term that means "of unknown cause." A common form of restrictive lung disease is "idiopathic interstitial pneumonitis." This means the patient has an inflammation of the lung (pneumonitis) that involves the connective tissue of the lung (interstitium) and is of unknown cause. But whether the cause is known or unknown, a diagnosis can be made and a treatment program started. Since scarring may occur, and scars cannot be reversed, an early diagnosis is important—before the scarring and other lung injuries become severe and irreversible.

Diseases of the blood vessels of the lung are less common. They develop because of injury to the small lung blood vessels or because blood clots (called emboli) block off the larger pulmonary vessels. Shortness of breath—developing sometimes suddenly, sometimes gradually—is usually the only symptom. Often these diseases go undiagnosed for long periods because patients "adapt" to their breathing limitations and therefore feel nothing is wrong. But, again, this is a mistake because early diagnosis and treatment are vital.

By far the most common lung diseases are of the obstructive type. That is why the rest of this book is devoted almost exclusively to them. Except for asthma, these diseases tend to cause shortness of breath mostly in people older than age 40—and this dyspnea is all too often attributed to age or being out of shape. Therefore, diagnosis is often long delayed because the individual does not seek medical attention.

OTHER BREATHING PROBLEMS

While shortness of breath, at rest or with activity, is the most common signal of lung disease, other problems may come before or after. Among the most frequent are cough, wheezing, chest pains, and spitting of blood.

Cough is, again, something we all experience. It requires your attention if it:

- Is persistent. Coughing day after day is not normal.
- Happens without an obvious cause (exposure to fumes, having "the flu").
- Produces yellow or green sputum.

The causes of cough range from sinusitis and chronic bronchitis to more serious things like tumors.

Wheezing—high-pitched noises coming from your throat or lungs—usually is due to mucus "stuck" somewhere in your windpipe or bronchial tubes. Lots of people may experience these noises after a viral infection. But if wheezing is persistent, has no obvious cause or is associated with shortness of breath, check it out. The causes range from viral infections to asthma to tumor.

Having chest pains—of any type—is not normal. However, many kinds of chest pains come from problems that are not serious, like muscle spasms or minor nerve pinches. But chest pains that are severe, or ones that persist, mean something—maybe something vital. The causes range widely: from heart attack to viral infections to blood clots reaching the lungs to mild rib injuries.

Coughing up blood, clearly, is not normal. If you cough up blood—even "little streaks"—something is wrong. But there are many causes for coughing up blood, from bronchitis and nasal congestion (the most common causes) to malignant tumors. The most common causes are not serious and can be easily treated. But seeing blood in what you cough up means you should act *immediately* to find out *why*.

THE CENTRAL POINTS

This brief summary of the breathing problems and their causes is far from comprehensive. Whole books can be written (and have been!) about any one of them. The central points are these:

- Shortness of breath (and other problems) may be a signal of disease.
- To determine whether it *is* such a signal ultimately requires evaluation by a doctor.
- Any of the breathing problems listed—if sudden in onset, severe, persistent and without an obvious cause—should be checked out. Chest pains and coughing up blood need prompt attention.
- A good history, physical examination, and simple laboratory tests can usually tell you and the doctor whether disease is present and, if so, what it is.
- Early diagnosis of all the diseases—including those of the lung—is important because delay in diagnosis means delay in treatment.
- Delay in treatment may lead to irreversible changes in the lungs (and, in some instances, in the heart as well).
- Of the lung diseases that cause shortness of breath, the "obstructive" ones are the most common.

This manual is primarily for individuals with obstructive lung disease, but some parts also apply to people with other kinds of lung diseases. If you have a lung disease other than asthma, chronic bronchitis, or emphysema, your doctor can tell you which parts of the book apply to you and which do not. Don't make a self-diagnosis. Proper understanding of your problem and its treatment begins with establishing a firm diagnosis. That is the doctor's job. Don't try to do it for him or her.

The Lungs: How They Are Put Together and How They Work

To understand your disease, you should know how normal lungs are constructed and how they work. Then it is easier to recognize what has happened to your lungs, why you get certain symptoms, and what you and your doctor can do to improve these symptoms. Some new vocabulary is involved. If you learn these new words, you will be able to talk with your doctor more easily and not be confused by things he/she says or articles you may read about lung disease.

HOW THE BODY'S ENGINE RUNS

The human body was designed to run on oxygen as its "energy" source, just as automobile engines run on gasoline or diesel fuel and power plants run on coal, oil, or other fuels. And, just as with other fuels, when the body "burns" oxygen for energy, waste products result; the two major waste products are water and carbon dioxide.

Therefore all of the body's functions depend on delivery of a steady supply of oxygen. Unfortunately, the body cannot store much oxygen. If delivery stops, the body "runs out of gas" (oxygen) within about 5 minutes. So the supply must be continuous, unlike the supply of food or water.

Furthermore, the waste products must be excreted promptly. Getting rid of water presents no problems. If the body retains water, it can still function and, sooner or later, excrete (get rid of) it through the kidneys as urine or through the sweat glands as perspiration. But if carbon dioxide builds up in the body, it creates acids in the blood. An excess of such acids can impair the function of important organs such as the brain and heart. And a build-up of carbon dioxide can produce symptoms such as headaches, drowsiness, and fatigue.

The lungs are designed to solve the twin problems of continuous oxygen delivery and carbon dioxide removal. They are the only route by which oxygen can be delivered to the body. Acids and carbon dioxide can be excreted by the kidneys, but the lungs get rid of carbon dioxide (and prevent acidity) much more quickly and efficiently than do the kidneys.

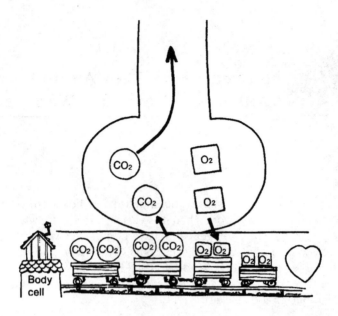

To carry out these two vital functions, the lungs need to have a practical way to bring fresh air (inspired air) into contact with the blood in a safe manner, so that the blood can pick up oxygen and get rid of excess carbon dioxide. Then the air must be efficiently expelled (expired) into the environment, and the blood pumped to the rest of the body.

HOW THE LUNGS ARE DESIGNED

Step One: Getting Air In and Out

This function is carried out by a system of branching air tubes (bronchial tubes) to bring air in and out of the lungs, and a system of blood tubes (pulmonary arteries) to bring blood to the lungs. The system of air tubes is called the *bronchial tree*, an appropriate name because it looks like an upside-down tree. It begins with a single, large tube (like the tree trunk) called the *windpipe* or *trachea*, which you can feel with your fingers in the front center of your neck. The trachea extends from the back of the mouth to the inside of the chest, or *thorax*. There the trachea divides into two major branches, one to the right lung, one to the left lung. Next, each of these main stem bronchi branches many times into smaller and smaller bronchial tubes, just as a tree branches. When the branches become very small (so small that they can be seen only with a microscope), they are given a new name: *bronchioles*. The larger bronchial tubes have cartilage in their walls. Cartilage is a rigid but flexible material—flexible enough to change shape as you breathe but rigid enough to prevent the larger bronchial tubes from collapsing. The smaller bronchial tubes have no cartilage in their walls; they are surrounded by a circle of muscle. If this muscle contracts, the tubes can be greatly nar-

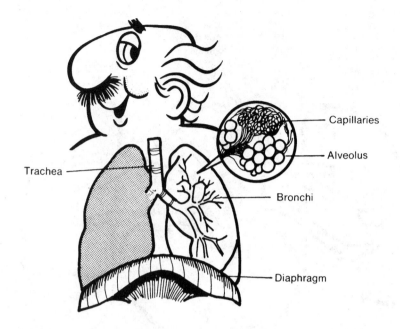

rowed. All bronchial tubes are lined by a delicate layer of cells and lubri-
cating liquid (the *mucous membrane*). Some of the cells in the membrane produce a sticky fluid called *mucus*, which coats the mucous membrane. Some
of the cells also have hair-like structures on them (*cilia*), which beat rhyth-
mically. The mucus lies on top of these cilia—a fact we will talk more about
later.

The bronchioles also branch, finally ending in a cluster of little bal-
loonlike structures called the *air sacs*, or *alveoli*. There are about 300 million
of these alveoli in the lungs. Thus one trachea leads to 300 million alveoli;
clearly, that involves a lot of branching! The alveoli have extremely thin
walls. They also contain "elastic" tissue in their walls, making them behave
much like tiny rubber balloons.

Step Two: Getting Blood In and Out

The system of blood tubes is similar in structure. It begins with one large
tube (*main pulmonary artery*) that comes out of the right side of the heart
(*right ventricle*). The main artery then splits into a right and left branch, one
supplying each lung. Then each of these branches, like those in the bronchial system, divides many times into smaller and smaller pulmonary arteries. The smallest branches of this system also get a new name: *arterioles*.
The arterioles run along the walls of the bronchioles. Finally, the arterioles
reach the alveoli; there they divide again into tiny vessels called *capillaries*.
The capillaries are in the walls of the alveoli. Therefore, the blood in the
capillaries is separated from the air in the alveoli only by the extremely

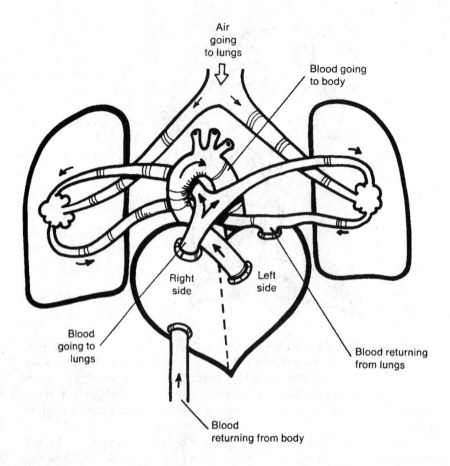

Air going to lungs

Blood going to body

Right side

Left side

Blood going to lungs

Blood returning from lungs

Blood returning from body

thin, elastic walls of the alveoli. This is why it is normally so easy for oxygen to get into, and carbon dioxide out of, the blood. There are about one billion capillaries—more than three for each air sac.

Once the blood has passed through the capillaries (and taken up new oxygen and disposed of excess carbon dioxide), it goes to the left side of the heart (*left atrium and ventricle*). The left ventricle now pumps this "fresh" blood to the organs of the body through the arteries. Therefore the arteries contain blood that has just come from the lungs. If the lungs are working properly, this blood contains normal amounts of oxygen and carbon dioxide; if they are not, the amounts of oxygen and carbon dioxide may be abnormal—the oxygen decreased and the carbon dioxide increased. That is why blood is often taken from arteries and analyzed; these *arterial blood gas values* tell your doctor how well your lungs are doing their job.

There is often confusion in people's minds about the "right side" and the "left side" of the heart. Although both sides are in one package (the heart) in your chest, you now know that the right heart pumps blood to the lungs; the left side receives this "fresh" blood and pumps it to the rest of the body. Therefore the right side of the heart can be directly affected by lung diseases. The left side is not. The blood in your arm or leg *veins* is returning to the right side of the heart to be pumped to the lungs. The veins are bluish and do not pulsate. Your arm or leg *arteries* contain blood that has just come from the lungs and is on its way to your organs (brain, kidneys, muscles, and so on). The *arteries* usually cannot be seen except as pulsations, but these pulsations are easily felt.

How the "Respiratory Pump" Works

There are a few more things you should know about how the lungs work. For example, what makes air go into (*inspiration*) and out of (*expiration*) the lungs? The elastic lungs are contained within an airtight box, the chest, or *thorax*. The chest is sealed at its lower end by the *diaphragm*, a thin muscle that separates the chest from the *abdomen* (stomach cavity). The diaphragm moves up and down like a piston. When it moves down (inspiration), the airtight thorax expands and a slight vacuum (negative pressure) is created. Air from the outside is therefore sucked into the lungs to overcome this vacuum. The elastic alveoli are

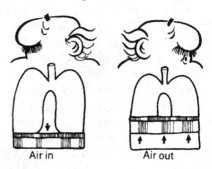

Air in   Air out

stretched, like expanding balloons; then the diaphragm relaxes and moves upward. The thorax becomes smaller, as do the elastic alveoli, which—again acting like balloons—expel the air from the lungs. For this system to work, it must be airtight so that a vacuum can be created during respiration. To ensure this airtight condition, the inner side of the chest wall and the outer side of the lungs are covered by a thin membrane (sheet of cells) called the *pleura*, which is moistened by a tiny amount of fluid so that the lungs slide smoothly when the thorax (chest wall) expands and contracts.

We are usually not aware of these things. Breathing normally goes on without our thinking about it, but as you know or will learn here, that is not the case if the lungs become abnormal. When the lungs become abnormal, muscles other than the diaphragm may be used to make the thorax larger and smaller. These are the intercostal muscles (which are between the ribs) and several muscles in the neck called *accessory muscles*. Usually, these muscles have little work to do during breathing; but in people with lung disease, they may have to do a great deal of work in breathing.

What "Controls" Breathing?

There is another thing that most of us do not think about when we breathe. How do we know how *much* to breathe? What controls *how deep* and *how fast* we breathe? Actually, we have a complicated "control" system built into the body that works a lot like a thermostat for regulating a central heating/cooling system. The usual thermostat registers temperature and turns the heater or air conditioner on or off to keep the temperature where you want it. The "breathing thermostat" senses the oxygen and carbon dioxide in the blood. It turns the breathing apparatus on and off (or makes it go faster or slower) to keep oxygen and carbon dioxide levels in the blood at proper levels. If the oxygen level in the blood falls, or if the carbon dioxide rises, this "thermostat" makes you breathe harder (more quickly and deeper). That is why, for example, when people go to high altitude, where there is less oxygen in the air, they breathe more quickly and deeply.

How the Lungs Are Protected

Finally, there are some things you should know about how the lungs protect themselves against impurities and other changes in the air we breathe. As you know, the air around us can be hot or cold and wet or dry, and can contain various irritating gases and particles. The lungs are rather delicate and work best when the air in them is *moist*, is at *body temperature* (37° C; 98.6° F), and is free of particles or irritating gases. Nature has designed several protective systems so that the lungs receive such air. The first of these systems is the *upper air passages*—the nose, the mouth, and the back of the mouth (*oropharynx*) where air entering the mouth or nose comes together. Above and around the nose and mouth are some "spaces" built into the skull; these spaces are called *sinuses*. These upper air passages and sinuses have two jobs: to regulate the temperature and wetness of the air you breathe in, and to remove irritating particles and gases from this air. If the system works, air entering your windpipe will be at just the right temperature and wetness and will be free of impurities. Thus the upper air passages can warm or cool inhaled air and can add or remove water from it; furthermore, irritant gases or particles are "trapped" in the mucus that coats these passages and are then removed by cough, sneeze, expectoration, or nose blowing.

If the upper air passages fail or are unable to do these things properly, air enters the lungs in less than optimal condition. The lungs themselves have several protection systems that then swing into action. The mucous membranes of the air tubes also are equipped to warm or cool air and to adjust its wetness. Particles or irritants can be "trapped" in the mucus that coats the bronchial tubes. After they are trapped, they can be coughed out or, more commonly, removed by a "mucus escalator" built into the lungs. There is a real "escalator" in the bronchial tree that consists of the mucous layer that is propelled from the small tubes to the windpipe by the *cilia* that beat toward the windpipe. This mucus is then either swallowed (without our being aware of it) or coughed out.

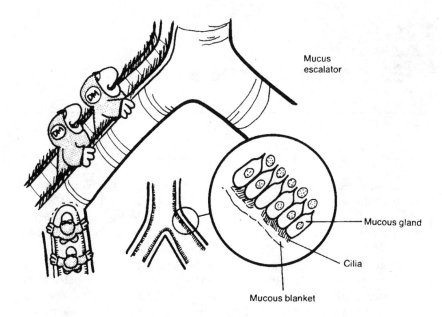

Of course, *cough* is another protection. Cough is produced by irritation of the bronchial tubes. This expels mucus much more rapidly than the "escalator." Cough also may alert us to the fact that we are inhaling irritating things and tell us to move away from them (if possible). Another "protection" is bronchial spasm. With severe irritation, the bronchial muscles contract, even in people without lung disease. This is the body's way of trying to protect us from inhaling irritants (by clamping down the small bronchial tubes). The sensation is an unpleasant one, but it may alert us to an irritant exposure from which we should escape.

Finally, some irritating gases or particles may defy these elaborate protective systems and get to the air sacs. Even then, another defense system exists—a special kind of white blood cells called *macrophages*. These cells wander through the air sacs searching for debris—viruses, bacteria, and particles that were inhaled. They engulf (suck up) such things, carry them off, and digest them. These cells cannot carry away *all* inhaled irritants. Some stay in the lungs and may cause irritation, future scarring, or other problems.

This, then, is the way normal lungs work and how they are constructed. Knowing about these things should help you to understand how to take care of your lungs and how, when they are injured or abnormal, to help them to work better.

3 COPD: What Does That Mean?

As has already been indicated, there are many lung diseases. The most common type of lung disease is obstructive lung disease. This is often referred to as COPD, which stands for Chronic Obstructive Pulmonary Disease. This term refers to a group of diseases that all share one common feature: difficulty in expelling air from the lungs. This is called *expiratory obstruction*.

There are three disease processes that are usually lumped together under the label of COPD: chronic bronchitis, emphysema, and asthma. Although each of these diseases develops in a different way, all cause expiratory obstruction. For patients, distinction among these three disorders is not critical because most individuals with COPD have some combination, and many of the symptoms and treatments are the same. (However, for research purposes, distinction among the COPDs remains important.)

CHRONIC BRONCHITIS

The problem in chronic bronchitis results from chronic inflammation and swelling of the cells lining the inside of the bronchi (air tubes). When in-

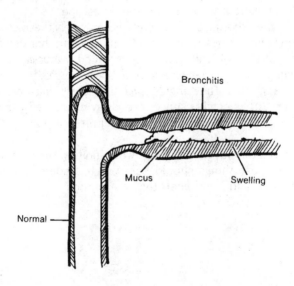

flamed, these cells produce excessive quantities of mucus. The swelling of these cells narrows the air tubes, making breathing more difficult. The excess mucus narrows the tubes further and even blocks some completely. The irritation and excess mucus often cause chronic cough in your body's attempt to expectorate the mucus. The lungs also become more easily infected because of these abnormalities. With repeated infections, lung damage may occur. Airways may become permanently dilated (*bronchiectasis*). Alveoli may become scarred (*fibrosis*). The narrowing of the bronchial tubes makes it more difficult for air to move into and out of them. If some of the tubes become blocked with mucus, the air sacs they supply cannot receive oxygen or get rid of carbon dioxide; they may, at least temporarily, collapse.

EMPHYSEMA

Emphysema is a disease in which the walls of the alveoli (air sacs) fracture (break). As these walls rupture, one large air sac replaces two, four, or many more small ones. The result is that the number of air sacs (alveoli) is reduced and many of those that remain are enlarged. One large sac is less elastic than the many tiny sacs were. Thus the patient with emphysema has *reduced elasticity* of the lungs. To visualize the problems this causes, think of how a balloon works. You must blow (work) to fill it. But when you stop blowing, the balloon recoils (deflates) without your doing anything. The balloon's own elasticity causes it to expel the air. This is how normal alveoli work. You work (inspire) to inflate them with air. But when you relax, the lungs recoil (deflate) without effort on your part. Expiration (blowing air out of the lungs) is therefore a passive event. It just happens.

In a person with emphysema the lungs and alveoli behave more like a paper bag. When you blow air into a paper bag, then stop blowing, what happens? Nothing. The bag stays full of air because it is nonelastic; it does

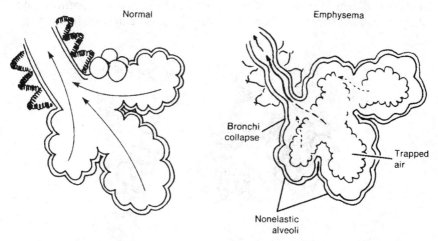

Normal

Emphysema

Bronchi collapse

Trapped air

Nonelastic alveoli

not recoil. To empty the air from a paper bag, you must squeeze it out—and you must expend effort to push the air out. People with emphysema must do the same thing: expend energy during expiration to squeeze air out of the lungs.

Furthermore, this loss of lung elasticity affects the smaller bronchial tubes. To push air out of these less elastic lungs, a higher pressure must be developed inside the chest. This higher pressure tends to collapse the smaller bronchial tubes, making it even harder to empty air from the alveoli. Worse expiratory obstruction results as the "neck of the balloon" (the bronchial tube) becomes narrowed. This tendency of the bronchial tubes to collapse also occurs with cough and makes it more difficult to cough up mucus. This collection of mucus, in turn, makes the lungs more susceptible to infection.

ASTHMA

The problem in asthma is that some irritant makes the muscles of the bronchial tubes go into spasm. This spasm narrows the bronchial tubes. Often this same irritant causes the lining cells of the bronchial tubes to swell and increase their production of mucus (secretions). These changes further narrow and clog up the bronchial tubes. When these things happen, the individual notices sudden shortness of breath and sometimes wheezing and cough.

There are several irritants that produce asthma. One is an *allergen*; that is, some material to which the patient is allergic. An allergy can show up as a rash, an upset stomach, or as bronchial spasm (asthma). Infection, cold air, smog, and cigarette smoke are other sources of irritation.

Many individuals with asthma have bronchial muscle that is more irritable than normal. Therefore, small amounts of inhaled irritants can cause bronchial spasm in these people but not in others. This "hyperirritability" of the bronchial tubes may run in families (that is, it may be inherited).

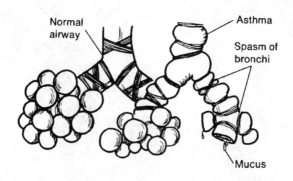

Normal airway

Asthma

Spasm of bronchi

Mucus

COPD: HOW DO YOU GET IT?

The causes of chronic obstructive lung disease have not been definitely determined. It is likely that the causes of emphysema, chronic bronchitis, and asthma are quite different. However, some features are common to each. For example, heredity seems to play a role in the tendency to develop each disorder.

Air pollution, occupational exposure to dust and fumes, and lung infections make all forms of COPD worse. Allergy plays a role in some cases of asthma but not in emphysema or bronchitis. Most of these things cannot be controlled by the affected person. But one factor is under the individual's control: cigarette smoking. Emphysema and chronic bronchitis rarely develop in nonsmokers; asthma is worsened by cigarette smoking.

COPD: WHAT ARE THE SYMPTOMS?

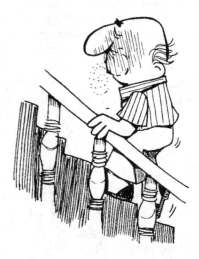

Usually the first thing a person with emphysema notices is shortness of breath on exertion (as when climbing stairs or walking quickly). As noted in Chapter 1, this symptom often is disregarded, and the individual feels it just means he or she is "out of shape" or "getting older." The first symptoms of chronic bronchitis are cough and mucus production. These symptoms are like a "chest cold" that hangs on week after week. Later, shortness of breath on exertion develops. The cough, mucus (sputum) production, and shortness of breath all may become suddenly worse if the individual develops the flu or some other type of lung infection.

Asthma usually starts with rather sudden attacks of cough, shortness of breath, and wheezing. These attacks may come and go at first. Many individuals with asthma have normal or near-normal lung function in between episodes. Later on, in some individuals, cough, mild wheezing, and shortness of breath may be present all the time (i.e., become chronic). The attacks may come on more frequently at certain times of the year (particularly spring or fall), or after exposure to known allergens or irritants, or only during exercise, or with onset of a cold. However, wheezing attacks also may appear without an obvious cause.

COPD: HOW DO YOU KNOW YOU HAVE IT?

The diagnosis of COPD involves many factors. The first step is for you to consult your doctor if you have any of the symptoms of COPD. The most common symptom is shortness of breath, particularly on exertion (walking up steps, carrying packages, hurrying during level walking). People often first notice that they can't "keep up" with their spouses or friends. A chronic 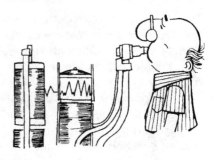 cough or wheezing may be other symptoms. However, problems *other than* COPD can cause similar symptoms. Trouble breathing, like pain in the chest, can mean many different things.

Your doctor will carry out a physical examination and other tests, such as pulmonary function tests, to determine whether you have COPD or some other problem. The pulmonary function tests usually include breathing into one or more machines that measure how well your lungs are working. Also, a small blood sample may be taken from an artery while you rest and during exercise to determine how well the lungs are delivering oxygen to the blood and removing carbon dioxide from it. A chest x-ray is taken to help this evaluation, but this alone cannot be used to diagnose COPD or other causes of lung symptoms. Using this evaluation as a basis, your doctor can

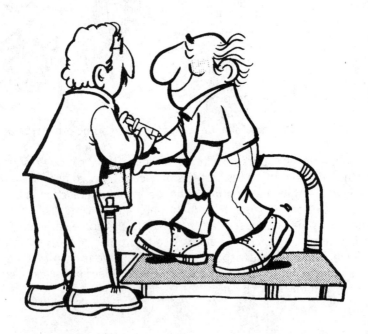

develop a proper treatment plan designed for you. The same tests can separate COPD from the other diseases that cause shortness of breath. So, no matter which kind of lung disease you have, the chest x-ray examination and pulmonary function tests provide valuable information.

COPD: WHAT CAN BE DONE ABOUT IT?

The most important factor in your treatment will be the relationship you have with your doctor. You must be willing to be frank and honest, and your doctor must be the same with you. Some parts of your treatment will be the doctor's responsibility, such as prescribing drugs, treatment, tests, and diets. A big part of the responsibility is yours. You must take the medicines as ordered, do your treatments at home, practice proper breathing, eat correctly, and most important of all, quit smoking if you haven't already. The treatment of COPD is a cooperative venture.

Each person's disease is different. Only your doctor knows which treatments and therapies are right for you. But only you know how you feel and how you respond to various treatments. Work with your doctor; ask questions. The more you know about your disease, the better off you are. The more your doctor knows about you, the better the treatment program that can be planned for you.

The treatment of COPD may include some or all of the following:

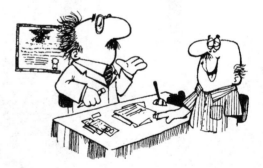

- Medications
- Good hydration (fluid intake)
- Proper breathing techniques
- Adequate diet
- Use of respiratory therapy
- Maintenance of muscle tone
- Graded physical activity
- Prevention and treatment of infections
- Use of supplemental oxygen in some cases
- Weight control
- Avoidance of allergens and/or irritants
- Bronchial drainage to remove excess mucus

The precise nature of your condition will determine the type of treatment prescribed. Sometimes very limited medication is all that is needed. Sometimes rather extensive treatment is required. The aims of treatment are to reverse the reversible, to preserve the function you have, to prevent complications, and to teach you how to use the function you have more efficiently. These aims can be achieved whether your problem is mild or severe.

COPD: WHAT IS YOUR RESPONSIBILITY?

Now that you have an understanding of what COPD means and the goals of treatment, it's time to add the most important ingredient—*you*. With enthusiasm, perseverance, and knowledge, you can play a major role in controlling your disease and alleviating some of your symptoms. The remainder of this manual is devoted to all aspects of treatment. After your doctor has outlined the various therapies he/she wants you to use, consult your manual for guidance and review.

4 Understanding Your Medications

Many people with lung disease take medications to improve their breathing and feel better. It is important to ask why the medication is prescribed, exactly how to take it, and what positive or negative reactions may occur. People are often afraid to take certain medications—and thus secretly don't take them. That is not in their best interest. A lot of wrong information is dispensed by friends, relatives, and people without medical training. Discuss each medicine with your doctor or pharmacist, both of whom can give you good information about all medications.

To treat the various types of lung diseases, different medications are used. Each medicine does a specific job to help the lungs function more effectively. Your doctor will determine which medications you need based on your history, the physical examination, the results of breathing tests, and other laboratory studies.

All medicines are chemicals. They may come from plant sources or from animals. Synthesized drugs are entirely human made. Medicines have their beneficial effects, but they may cause side effects. A medicine taken by mouth must enter the stomach and then the blood in order to reach the lungs. Not only can medicines upset the stomach, but they pass through many other organs while on their way to the lungs and may exert these other effects, called side effects. Most of the time these effects are well tolerated and may disappear with time. You should be familiar with what your medicine is supposed to do and also with its side effects.

Another important fact to remember is that each medicine has two names: a generic (chemical) name and a brand (company) name. The generic name is always the same for each drug, no matter which company manufactures it. The brand name for a drug is the property of the company that markets that drug. In some states it is possible for your pharmacist to substitute a less expensive generic brand drug for the more expensive branded product. Some-times the practice may cause you some confu-   sion and you may think you have received the wrong prescription. If there are any questions because the pills look different to you, consult with your pharmacist. Besides providing you with medicines, many pharmacies provide other helpful services. For example, many pharmacists maintain a complete record of all prescriptions you have received from any physician, dentist, or other doctor. This "patient profile" can then be reviewed periodically by the pharmacist for drug interactions, a situation that occurs when two or more drugs taken at the same time work against each other. Ask your pharmacist or physician to explain this in more detail.

After each category of medication that follows, list (with the help of your physician, pharmacist, or nurse) the names of the medications you take, along with the dose and time schedule for each drug.

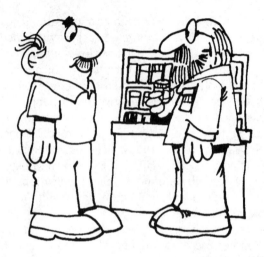

BRONCHODILATORS

Bronchodilators relax the muscles of the breathing tubes, making them wider and allowing air to get in and out more easily. Bronchodilators can be taken as pills, liquids, or aerosol sprays (see Chapter 5). The most common of these drugs are theophylline (a xanthine), adrenergic (adrenaline-like) drugs, and anticholinergic (atropine-like) drugs. There are many different preparations of these types of drugs, and new ones appear regularly. Newer medications tend to be safer, easier to use, and more selective in their effects. As with all medicines, there may be side effects. Xanthine drugs may cause an upset stomach and heartburn. Adrenergic drugs, depending on the form taken (pill or spray) and on how much you use, can increase your heart rate, make you feel jittery or nervous, or cause muscle tremors. Inhaled forms of adrenergic and anticholinergic drugs tend to be better tolerated than oral or other types.

STEROIDS

Steroid drugs are all "relatives" of the hormone *cortisol*, which the body produces normally. These corticosteroids help to dilate the bronchial tubes, decrease the swelling of bronchial tube lining, and decrease lung inflammation. Steroids also have many potential side effects. They may make you feel very energetic and give you a (false) sense of well-being. Other common side effects include weight gain, redistribution of fat, easy bruising, stomach irritation, and cataracts in the eyes. The side effects depend on the dose of the drug taken, how you take it (pill or spray), and the length of time you take it. You must never discontinue oral steroids yourself or alter the dose without your physician's advice. People often hear stories about the side effects of steroids—stories that worry them. Remember that the side effects relate to the amount and the time schedule of any drug you take. Steroids are no different. And, like any drug, your doctor prescribes them only when you need them and in the amounts you require. For many years, steroids were available only by pill or injection. Now certain special steroids can be inhaled as an aerosol, directly into the lungs. Inhaled steroids are absorbed very slowly and poorly into the blood. Therefore they have beneficial effects on the lungs while causing fewer side effects. For people who need only small doses of steroids, these inhalations may replace oral steroids. However, all steroids must be taken on a regular schedule because they do not give immediate effects; so they are not to be used as you "need" them, but regularly, to *prevent* symptoms. Remember, these are potent medicines and must be taken only as directed by your physician.

CROMOLYN SODIUM

Cromolyn sodium is a medication used mainly by patients who have asthma. It is taken by inhalation and works only to *prevent* symptoms and bronchospasm. To do this, it must be taken regularly. It should never be used during an asthmatic attack, because it can actually make an attack worse.

DIGITALIS

Digitalis is the generic, overall name for heart pills that strengthen the heart muscle. These drugs make the heart beat more slowly and with more force. Most patients with lung disease do not have heart problems that require digitalis, but some do. Digitalis drugs must be used carefully. The dose should never be changed without your doctor's order.

EXPECTORANTS

The purpose of expectorants is to liquefy secretions and make them easier to cough up.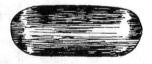
Generally, they are used only by patients with very heavy bronchial secre-

tions. Their value is debated, with no conclusive medical opinion as to whether they work or not. The most widely used expectorants are potassium iodide (SSKI) and glycerol guaiacolate (GG). Potassium iodide can cause a rash and swelling of the salivary glands because of allergies to iodide. Newer types of expectorants have been developed and are being evaluated.

ANTIBIOTICS

Antibiotic medications are used to help fight bacterial infections. There are many different types that are used against different bacteria. Some are given as pills or capsules, others by injection. Penicillin, sulfa drugs, tetracycline, and erythromycin are generic names of some of the drugs in this category that are commonly used for patients with lung diseases. You should take these drugs in the exact dose and at the time specified by your doctor, who will tell you what side effects may occur. For example, an upset stomach or bowel problems are common side effects with certain antibiotics. You must always finish the course of antibiotic therapy that your physician prescribes, even when you feel better after only a few doses.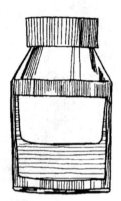

DIURETICS

Diuretics (water pills) help rid your body of excess fluid. This fluid retention, called *edema*, usually shows up as swollen ankles and legs. There are many reasons why edema may develop in patients with lung disease. Your doctor will provide you with guidelines on the use of the drugs that treat edema. Overuse of diuretics can make you weak and should be avoided (see Potassium Supplements).

POTASSIUM SUPPLEMENTS

When diuretics are taken regularly, they cause loss of not only fluid but also potassium. This may result in weakness and leg cramps. Potassium supplements are given to counteract these effects.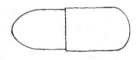
Eating high-potassium foods is sometimes sufficient to replenish lost potassium (see Chapter 12).

MOOD ELEVATORS

Mood elevating drugs are designed to help you feel less depressed. People with chronic health problems often have periods of feeling "blue." If this feeling persists, you should consult your doctor or a psychiatrist for help in dealing with this problem.

TRANQUILIZERS AND SEDATIVES

Tranquilizers and sedatives are designed to calm or relax you and to help you sleep. These drugs can dangerously depress your breathing if taken in excess. Never increase the dose without consulting your doctor. Some symptoms (such as insomnia or irritability) may mean that your lungs are not working properly and that sedatives and tranquilizers should be decreased, not increased. Your physician knows when and how to adjust the dose of these drugs.

FLU AND PNEUMONIA VACCINES

Vaccines help you to fight off serious viral (flu) infections and certain bacterial (pneumococcal) infections. A new flu vaccine is prepared each year and is usually available in the fall before the start of the flu season. The pneumococcal vaccine needs to be given only once.

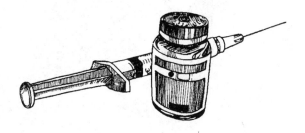

OXYGEN

Sometimes patients with lung disease cannot transfer enough oxygen from the alveoli to the blood; therefore the amount of oxygen in the blood falls below normal levels. A low blood oxygen level impairs the body's engine (see Chapter 2). Whatever the reason for the oxygen lack, the treatment is the same: take a drug that overcomes the deficiency. In the case of oxygen deficit, that "drug" is oxygen.

Like all drugs, oxygen is prescribed by your doctor. The drugs you take for your respiratory problem are ordered by your doctor in a specific amount, at specific times, by a specific route. For example, aminophylline (drug), 250 mg. (dose), four times a day (times), by mouth (route). Likewise, oxygen is prescribed by your doctor in the same manner: oxygen (drug), 2 liters/minute (dose), during exercise (time), by nasal cannula (route). Your doctor determines the appropriate dose based on blood oxygen level measurements taken at rest and while exercising. As with other drugs, you must not increase or decrease your oxygen flow without the doctor's advice. Turning the liter flow above the prescribed dose may cause serious complications.

Remember that millions of dollars each year are spent on medicines. You can help make the most of your medicine dollars by taking your medications as prescribed and communicating problems with your doctor. Each person should receive those medicines that are best for him or her. Those that are good for you may not necessarily be good for your friend or relative!

5 Oxygen and Aerosols: What They Can Do for You

Many people with chronic lung disease are treated with some type of respiratory therapy equipment or hear about such equipment from others. Often it is first used during an emergency room visit or stay in the hospital. Sometimes it is introduced during a pulmonary rehabilitation program.

Respiratory therapy equipment comes in various sizes, with various degrees of complexity and varying costs. Some devices can be helpful in delivering inhaled medications that may improve symptoms such as wheezing, shortness of breath, and coughing. Equipment can be used to supply oxygen therapy that can be useful for people with low blood oxygen levels (a condition termed *hypoxemia*). The indications for and proper use of equipment should be determined by your physician. A respiratory therapist or nurse can help you to better understand the use and care of your equipment. Individual needs vary greatly; there is no single treatment plan that applies to all people with chronic lung disease. The device that gave you so much relief in the hospital or in the doctor's office may present some problems for you at home and may not be of value there. Often you can do

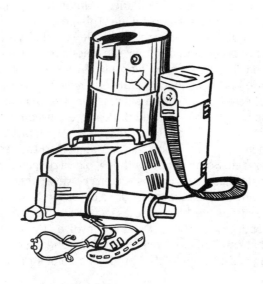

things yourself that will help your breathing more than a machine can. There is no substitute for being informed about your disease.

If you do need equipment at home, the simplest device that will do the job is the best choice. **Remember: The more complex the equipment, the bigger your commitment is for its use, care, and maintenance.** To achieve maximal benefits, you should clearly understand the purpose and correct usage of the equipment prescribed for you.

Also, be aware that cost is not a good measure of the value of a device. Inexpensive devices are often as effective as costly ones. Fancy dials and gadgets are no indication that you are getting "the best." Your doctor, respiratory therapist, or nurse should be familiar with these devices and will indicate whether you need them and which best suits your condition.

The devices most frequently used for home care can be conveniently grouped into two categories: oxygen therapy and aerosol therapy. This chapter describes the equipment associated with the delivery of oxygen as "oxygen therapy equipment" and the devices that produce visible mist for inhalation as "aerosol therapy equipment." You may also need a combination of these treatments.

OXYGEN THERAPY

What is oxygen? It is an element, a drug, and a gas. Every cell in the body needs energy to function. Cells get their energy from a combination of the food we eat plus oxygen. This energy enables us to use our muscles to breathe, to perform work, and to carry out all bodily functions.

To be useful, air that contains oxygen is inhaled and travels through air passages to alveoli (air sacs) in the lungs, where it then moves across into small blood vessels called capillaries. Carbon dioxide is a gas that is eliminated from our bodies as we exhale. This process by which the body takes in oxygen and eliminates carbon dioxide is called *gas exchange*. If gas exchange does not occur normally, then the amount of oxygen in your blood can be decreased. There are many reasons why some people with chronic lung disease have low oxygen levels while others do not. For example, when the lungs are affected by a disease such as emphysema, air may not flow well to all areas because of damaged or destroyed alveoli. In such areas of the lung, the blood in the capillaries may not be completely replenished with fresh oxygen. Then the blood that is pumped to the rest of the body will be low in oxygen. Some people with low blood oxygen levels may show signs of blue nail beds, ears, or lips. Often, however, there are no visible signs, which is why an assessment by your physician is so important.

Oxygen levels in the blood are assessed by two methods: oximetry and arterial blood gases (ABGs). Oximetry involves the use of a machine and a sensor that can be placed over the skin on the finger or the ear lobe to measure oxygen saturation. This method is helpful for monitoring trends without obtaining a blood sample. Oximetry is often used in doctors' offices, clinics, and in your home by oxygen equipment. The other method, measuring arterial blood gases, involves drawing blood from an artery, often in the wrist area. Specially maintained equipment and trained technicians are needed to obtain and process the blood sample. This method tends to be more accurate and provides additional information, such as the carbon dioxide level in the blood.

Oxygen therapy may be prescribed when an individual has been assessed with either one of these methods. It is prescribed only when oxygen levels in the blood are low and need to be increased to a more normal level to support the body's needs. Oxygen therapy is not prescribed for shortness of breath or fatigue. There are many reasons why patients with chronic lung disease can become short of breath without having low oxygen levels. No recommended standard exists for how often an arterial blood gas or oximetry test should be performed. This is at the discretion of your physician. However, many health insurers require an annual test to continue coverage for oxygen prescriptions.

What if your body is not getting enough oxygen? It is known that blood vessels often constrict (narrow) when oxygen levels are low. The right side of the heart must work harder to pump blood through these narrowed blood vessels. The result can be an increased strain on the right side of the heart. For this and other reasons, medical studies have shown that people with low oxygen levels live longer and better lives if they use oxygen than if they do not.

If your blood oxygen levels are low, your physician will prescribe supplemental oxygen for you. If you use oxygen therapy, as for any drug, it is essential to have a prescription. The prescription should tell you when to use the oxygen and how much to use. Many people with chronic lung disease have prescriptions that direct them to use one amount at rest and sleep and a higher amount with activity. Others use oxygen only with physical activity. It is important to keep in mind that being out of breath does not necessarily mean that you have a low blood oxygen level. The only way to be certain is to be assessed by medical professionals with an arterial blood gas or oximetry test.

Oxygen makes up 21% of the air around us. Oxygen can be extracted from the air by a very special industrial process that yields 100% oxygen that has been purified and dehumidified. Once extracted, oxygen is packaged and made available for home delivery.

A wide variety of systems are available for home use. Oxygen equipment can be rented or purchased; the oxygen comes as compressed gas or as a liquid. You can also purchase or rent electrical devices that concentrate oxygen from room air. Some oxygen systems are portable; some are not. The choice of oxygen sources is broader than ever before and continues to improve.

OXYGEN EQUIPMENT

Sources of Oxygen

There are three sources of oxygen available for use in the home: compressed gas, liquid oxygen, and oxygen concentrators.

COMPRESSED GAS: TANKS AND CYLINDERS

This is the oldest method for storing oxygen. The oxygen gas is compressed and stored in tanks or cylinders constructed of either steel or aluminum. Aluminum tanks tend to be lighter in weight and more portable. Tanks come in many sizes. Large stationary ones are often placed in the bedroom; smaller ones are used for exercising or traveling outside the home. For safety reasons, cylinders must be secured upright with a stand or a cart, which is supplied with the oxygen.

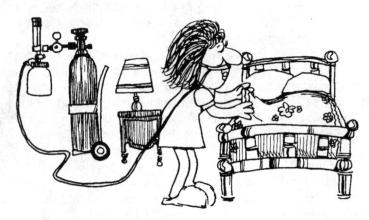

LIQUID OXYGEN

Liquid oxygen is widely used for people who lead active life-styles. A cooling process is utilized to change the oxygen from a gas to a liquid. The advantage of liquid oxygen is that it takes up less space than the gas form. Therefore, liquid oxygen can be stored in smaller, more convenient containers. However, it cannot be stored for long periods because it evaporates. Liquid oxygen also requires care in handling.

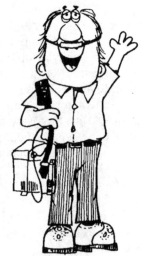

OXYGEN CONCENTRATOR

An oxygen concentrator is an electrical unit about the size of a nightstand or end table. The concentrator "makes its own oxygen" by removing the oxygen molecules from room air. Advantages of this method of oxygen therapy are that it may be less expensive in the long run, it does not require refilling or replacing tanks, and it can be easier to manage. However, there are also disadvantages. Oxygen concentrators are not portable, which means that if you are using oxygen 24 hours a day, a portable system such as a small oxygen tank will be needed for use outside of your home. Using the oxygen concentrator may also increase your electric bill (even though most gas and electric companies offer reduced rates for life-supporting equipment, provided you register with them); it also may be noisy and give off heat. Back-up cylinders are required in the event of a power failure. If you use a high flow rate, this method may not be adequate because the actual percentage of oxygen inspired may drop as the flow rate increases.

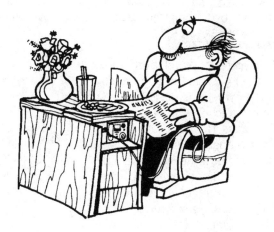

Safety and Storage

Oxygen is a relatively safe gas, but because it supports combustion, it must be handled with caution. Oxygen itself does not burn, but it aids in igniting combustible materials. For example, any spark or open flame expands considerably, like a "flash-fire." Also, oxygen in tanks is under high pressure; therefore, if the top of the tank is knocked loose, the tank can "take off" like a rocket. Liquid oxygen is very cold, and touching the "steam" that may escape can "burn" you.

Remember

- The room in which oxygen is stored should be dry, cool, and well ventilated; keep oxygen away from heat, flame, and spark sources.
- Be certain that the oxygen tank is fastened securely. This will prevent it from being knocked over.

- Avoid inhaling the irritating debris that may accumulate at the bottom of cylinders by always changing cylinders when the pressure regulator reads 500 psi (pounds per square inch).
- Never permit grease, oil, or any other potential combustible substance to come into contact with oxygen delivery equipment.
- Smoking is not permitted within 10 feet of a source from which oxygen is being administered. Also, there must be at least 10 feet between the oxygen source and any open flame or possible source of electrical sparks.

Oxygen Delivery Devices

NASAL CANNULA

Most commonly, a nasal cannula is the appliance used to deliver low concentrations of oxygen for extended periods. The cannula is a hollow, light plastic device with two small extensions; one enters each nostril. The cannula is kept in place by looping the attached tubing over the ears.

TRANSTRACHEAL CATHETER

Transtracheal oxygen is a relatively new method for delivering oxygen in a more efficient manner. The catheter is placed directly into the windpipe (trachea) through a small incision in the neck. This is usually done through a minor outpatient surgical procedure. Since the oxygen is delivered directly into the lungs, rather than through the nose, the flow rate of oxygen frequently can be reduced; this allows the oxygen source to last longer, a distinct advantage for portable systems. In addition, better oxygenation can be 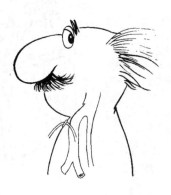 achieved for individuals who require high flow rates (such as 4 liters per minute or more). Other possible advantages include more continuous therapy (the catheter stays in place at all times), more comfort and convenience, better cosmetic appearance, and fewer problems related to having the nasal cannula on the patient's face. However, use of the transtracheal catheter also requires regular care and cleaning and more problem solving by the patient. Appropriate patient and caregiver training must be provided.

OXYGEN CONSERVING DEVICES

In addition to transtracheal oxygen therapy, other new devices have been developed to reduce the oxygen flow requirement and extend the period of time a particular gas source will last. "Reservoir" nasal cannulas provide for storage of oxygen during exhalation in reservoirs located either near the nasal prongs or in a pendant located around the neck. Other devices, called "demand" devices, either attach to the oxygen source or are built into the

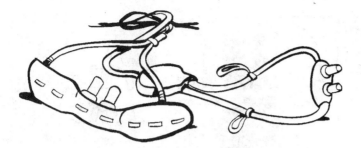

system. Demand devices turn the flow of oxygen *on* with inspiration (when you "demand" it) and *off* with expiration, so that less oxygen is wasted.

Additional Equipment for Oxygen Therapy

A compressed gas cylinder has a regulator and flowmeter attached to it. The regulator is a device that reduces the high pressure of the oxygen as it leaves the cylinder. A dial on the regulator also tells you how much oxygen is in the cylinder: a full tank of oxygen usually contains 2200 psi pressure. As you use oxygen, the pressure reading will decrease. If you use liquid oxygen, the contents are determined by weighing the container with a scale that comes with the container or by reading the contents dial (e.g., ½ full, ¼ full, empty).

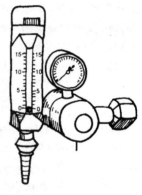

   The flowmeter is a measuring device or dial; it is paired with the oxygen regulator if you are using compressed gas or is attached to your liquid oxygen container or concentrator. Never use oxygen without a flow control. The flowmeter regulates how much oxygen is delivered in the liters per minute prescribed for you by your doctor.

   A humidifier is a bottle or jar filled with water and attached to an oxygen flowmeter. The purpose of the humidifier is to replace water vapor that has been removed from oxygen during the manufacturing process.

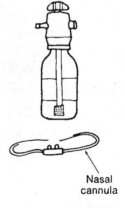

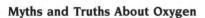

Nasal cannula

Myths and Truths About Oxygen

Myth: Oxygen is addicting. Once you start it, you will have to use it forever.

Truth: Oxygen is not addicting. Supplemental oxygen is needed only when your own lungs cannot supply enough. If you no longer need it, you can stop using it.

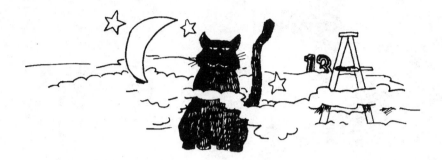

Myth: If a little oxygen is good, a lot of oxygen is better.

Truth: Oxygen is a drug. Use it only as instructed. Like any other drug, too much can be harmful.

Myth: Shortness of breath means lack of oxygen, so if you become short of breath, you should take oxygen.

Truth: Shortness of breath is not always associated with the lack of oxygen. There are many other causes for shortness of breath. Working hard to breathe, as can occur in many chronic lung diseases, can make you short of breath even if there is plenty of oxygen in your blood. Only by testing the level of oxygen in your blood can your doctor tell if you need supplemental oxygen.

Myth: People who need to use oxygen must be confined to their home and can't do anything.

Truth: People who use oxygen can lead a normal life. Several types of portable oxygen systems are available. With good planning, you can be active and mobile.

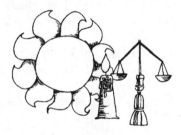

Think Ahead: Things to Consider Before You Select a Home Oxygen System

1. Ask your doctor, respiratory therapist, or nurse to recommend a practical system for your needs and life-style.

2. Ask your doctor to refer you to a reputable medical equipment supplier.

3. Compare portable systems for cost, weight, size, duration of oxygen supply, and refilling capabilities.

4. If an oxygen concentrator is recommended, compare size, noise levels, and monthly electrical cost. If you use a concentrator, be sure to register with your gas and electric company to keep electric costs down.

5. Find out whether the system you select is approved by your medical insurance carrier and whether they will reimburse you for all or part of the cost. Often the medical equipment company will assist you.

6. Obtain written instructions from your physician or equipment supplier for the correct use of your oxygen system. Make sure you understand these instructions.

7. Learn how to determine the number of hours of oxygen each source will provide. Keep enough on hand. Arrange deliveries on a regular schedule so you won't run out at night or during a weekend.

8. Ask a family member or friend to assist you in making the equipment selection and in learning about its use and safety.

AEROSOL THERAPY

The respiratory therapy devices discussed here are those associated with aerosol or "mist" therapy. This treatment modality involves the inhalation of medications directly into the air passages of the lungs. Inhaling medications is a relatively fast and reliable method for symptom relief. Chest congestion with thick secretions and wheezing may be improved with the inhalation of medications.

Metered Dose Inhaler

The metered dose inhaler (MDI) is a very simple, easy-to-handle, and convenient mode for inhalation of medications. It consists of a small cartridge that may contain various types of medicine, chiefly bronchodilators or steroids (see Chapter 4), and a mouthpiece for dispensing the drug. The advantage of this type of aerosol therapy is its portability, safety, and minimal care, as well as its quick action.

INSTRUCTIONS FOR METERED DOSE INHALER

1. Assemble metered dose inhaler for use. Shake well.

2. Exhale through pursed lips to a comfortable level (see Chapter 6).

3. Place the open end of the mouthpiece into your open mouth past the front teeth, as shown in the figure at the right.

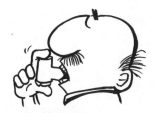

4. Do not close your lips—this allows more air to be inhaled through the mouth to aid in carrying the medication deeper into your lungs.

5. As you start taking a slow deep breath, press down firmly one time on the cartridge to release the medication.

6. Hold your breath a few seconds to allow the medication to settle on the surface of your airways. (This will prevent you from exhaling the medication and will aid in obtaining relief.)

7. Exhale slowly, using pursed lips.

8. Repeat only as prescribed; rest a minute or so before taking additional puffs, if prescribed.

9. Keep the MDI clean and free from dirt and lint by placing it in a clean plastic bag.

10. Wash and disinfect the plastic mouthpiece dispenser regularly (at least weekly).

11. Date MDI cartridges when you begin using them. Check the amount of medication in your MDI using the "float test" so that you may obtain refills ahead of time. An easy way to estimate how much medication is left inside is to place the cartridge in a container of water and observe its position as it floats.

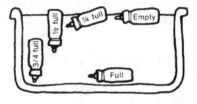

Note: Do not overuse. Use only as directed by your doctor.

Spacers and Extenders

Spacers and extenders are chambers placed between you and your metered dose inhaler. They allow the medication to be released first into the chamber before you inhale it. The primary advantage is to simplify the *timing* of medication release, which is so important in using the metered dose inhalers. Spacers and extenders may also help those who experience coughing spasms when using an inhaler. In addition, they help to deliver more of the medication into the lungs and less into the mouth and throat. If your phy-

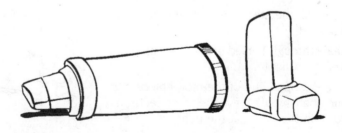

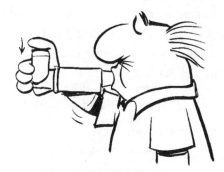

sician prescribes a spacer or extender for you, make sure that you receive instructions for use, replacement, and cleaning of the device.

Nebulizers: The Mini-Neb and the Ultrasonic

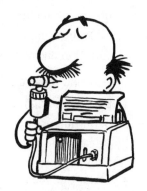

A nebulizer is a device that is designed to produce a mist or fog from a liquid; it can be powered either by pressurized air, by oxygen, or by an electrical source.

A very popular setup for aerosol therapy at home is the "mini-neb" and air compressor. This system is compact, is simple to operate, and requires little maintenance. It is used primarily to deliver medications or moisture for short periods of time, two to four times throughout the day. The maximum capacity of a small nebulizer is approximately 15 ml (1 tablespoon).

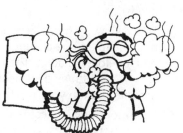

The ultrasonic nebulizer is a very effective nebulizer that operates from an electrical source. This unit transforms electrical energy into vibrations, which are then transferred to a liquid. Vibration of the liquid results in a fine, dense, cool mist. This device can be more expensive than conventional nebulizers.

IMPORTANT INFORMATION TO KNOW ABOUT AEROSOL THERAPY

1. The name of the equipment you are using and its parts
2. How often you should use it (for example, twice a day), and for how long (for example, 20 minutes)
3. What solutions to put in the nebulizer
4. How you should prepare, store, and measure the solutions you are using

5. What parts of the nebulizer unit should be removed for cleaning

6. How to clean and disinfect your nebulizer (must be done every 24 hours)

7. How to troubleshoot minor malfunctions

8. **Most important:** the correct breathing pattern to use while taking aerosol therapy (we recommend slow, deep breathing and a slight pause after full inspiration to allow the liquid particles to settle in the lungs)

CHECK POINTS BEFORE EACH TREATMENT

1. Be sure tubing and accessories are clean and dry.

2. Be sure the equipment set-up is properly connected to your machine.

3. Place the correct dose of medication in the nebulizer cup.

    a. Use a clean measuring device.

    b. Cap all medication bottles after use.

    c. Pour saline solution or water directly into the nebulizer cup.

4. Turn the machine on and check for mist production at the mouthpiece.

TAKING YOUR TREATMENT

1. Sit in an upright position. Relax.

2. Set a timer or check your watch before starting.

3. Be sure the nebulizer is in an upright position and the tubes are not bent or kinked.

4. Place the mouthpiece between your teeth and bite gently, keeping your lips tight around it so air does not escape. (A nose clip may be needed.)

5. Take a slow, moderately deep breath, letting the air and medication from the machine fill your lungs. After inspiring, pause (hold breath 1-2 seconds) before exhaling. Then exhale slowly. Always remember to breathe slowly. Sometimes treatments help to bring up sputum or phlegm. Don't hesitate to stop your treatment to cough this out.

6. Your mouth may become dry during or after a treatment. You may stop your treatment for a drink of water.

AFTER YOUR TREATMENT

1. After each treatment, disassemble and rinse the nebulizer and mouthpiece. Shake off the excess water and place these parts on a clean paper towel. Cover with another paper towel until your next treatment.

2. After the last treatment of the day, follow your doctor's instructions for cleaning and disinfecting the equipment.

CARE AND CLEANING OF YOUR RESPIRATORY EQUIPMENT

You must take proper care of all equipment that delivers mists or medications into your lungs. If your equipment becomes contaminated with bacteria, even your own bacteria, you can infect yourself and put an extra strain on your lungs and heart. Be sure you clearly understand what equipment parts need to be washed and disinfected. Ask your doctor, therapist, or equipment rental company to recommend an effective technique and disinfecting agent. (We recommend daily cleaning for any mist-producing equipment.)

The following instructions offer a simple approach that is used frequently.

Supplies Needed

Liquid detergent (such as dishwashing liquid)

White vinegar or commercially available disinfectant

Soft brush

Two basins (do not use sink)

1. Basin 1 should contain detergent water (discard daily)

2. Basin 2 should hold one part vinegar to one part water (discard every other day; cover between use). If other disinfectants are used, they should be mixed and discarded according to the manufacturer's instruction.

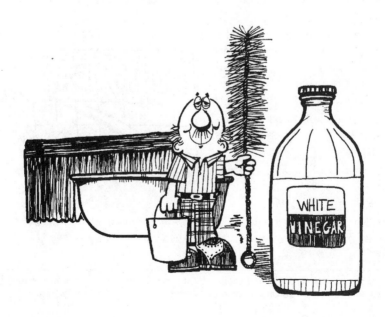

The Routine for Cleaning

1. Remove all washable parts of equipment and disassemble.
2. Wash in warm water with detergent (basin 1). Scrub all parts gently with brush. Cleaning removes medication residues, secretions, or any foreign materials.
3. Rinse thoroughly under running tap water.
4. Soak equipment in disinfecting solution (basin 2) for a minimum of 30 minutes if using vinegar or according to manufacturer's instructions if using another disinfectant (to kill bacteria). Be sure hollow parts are filled with solution and equipment is completely submerged.
5. Rinse completely under hot tap water; be careful not to let your equipment touch the sink.
6. Air-dry your equipment as follows:
   a. Shake or swing excess water out of tubing and hard-to-dry areas of accessories.
   b. Hang tubing to allow it to drip completely dry.*
   c. Place all other pieces of equipment on clean paper towels and cover with clean paper towels.

Remember

1. Discard detergent solution (basin 1) daily.
2. Vinegar solution (basin 2) should be covered and can be kept for 2 days, but no longer. Store in a clean area.
3. Wipe down all surfaces of the machine with a clean damp cloth daily. Then cover and store the machine in a clean area between treatments.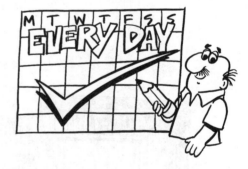
4. Use the scrub brush and basins only for cleaning *this equipment*.
5. Store dry tubing and accessories in new sealed plastic bags.
6. Have two complete sets of washable equipment so you always have a clean, dry set-up available for use the following day.

---

*If you choose not to clean the nebulizer tubing, replace it often, whenever the tubing becomes hard to pinch (less pliable) or sticky when touched and when discoloration occurs.

7. Hair dryers or blowers are not to be used to dry equipment.
   All equipment must be washed as stated every 24 hours!

How to Prepare Sterilized Water or Normal Saline for Home Use

Here are instructions for making your own solutions for inhalation. It may be less expensive for you to prepare them than to buy them. However, it may be more convenient to purchase prepared normal saline (a mild salt solution) to use with your medication. Remember that bacteria can grow in your solutions unless you are extremely careful. Please follow these instructions exactly as they are written.

1. You need a jar with a lid that fits snugly. A small jam jar or juice bottle will do.

2. Thoroughly wash this jar and its lid in detergent; rinse.

3. Place the jar and its lid in a clean pan and fill with tap water so that the jar is completely submerged. Place a lid on the pan and gently boil the jar for 15 minutes to sterilize it.

4. After you have boiled the jar, pour the tap water out of the pan. (Use the pan lid to prevent the sterilized jar from falling out.)

5. After the jar and lid have cooled, remove them from the pan. Place them upright on a clean counter. Do not let anything "unsterile" touch the insides of the jar or lid. Do not dry them with a towel or place them upside down to drain.

6. Resterilize the jar and lid at least once each week.

7. Pour distilled water (twice the desired amount) into the clean pan used to boil the jar. If preparing normal saline (salt water), add ¼ teaspoon of salt to every 2 cups of distilled water.

8. Boil gently for 15 minutes. You will have about half the water you started with. Let the water cool and then pour it into the "sterile" jar; cover it with the "sterile" lid.

9. Store this in the refrigerator. Discard any unused solutions at least once a week.

10. To remove any solution from the jar, pour directly into your nebulizer. Never place an "unsterilized" eyedropper, teaspoon, or other measuring device into the solution in the jar. Do not pour any extra solution back into the jar once it has been removed—discard it.

Saline or diluent solutions may be purchased from pharmacies in cans without a prescription or in pre-packaged vials that require a prescription. These may be more expensive, but they are convenient and provide accurately measured doses.

6 The Art of Better Breathing and Coughing

BREATHING EXERCISES

In obstructive lung diseases like COPD, airways can collapse when you exhale and trap stale air in the air sacs. When this happens, your lungs are full of stale air and there isn't enough room for you to breathe in fresh air.

Pursed Lip Breathing

The pursed lip breathing technique (pursed lips means having your lips in a whistling or kissing position) will help you remove stale trapped air from your lungs. This will make room for a fresh breath of oxygenated air and reduce your shortness of breath. Pursed lip breathing provides a resistance to exhaled air at the mouth and maintains a higher pressure in the airways. This keeps the airways open longer 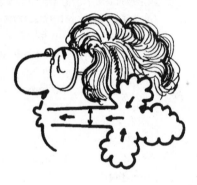 so that you can squeeze with your abdominal muscles and push more air out.

1. Inhale through your nose with your mouth closed.
2. Exhale through your mouth with your lips pursed.

Normal movement of the diaphragm

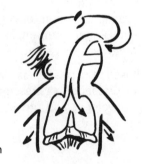

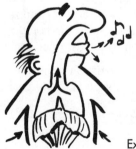

Inhalation

Exhalation

3. Contract your abdominal muscles, squeezing inward and upward against your diaphragm and compressing lungs to get the stale air out.

4. Make your exhalation at least twice as long as your inhalation (for example, "in 2," "out 2, 3, 4"). You may want to spend more time breathing out (for example, "in 2," "out, 2, 3, 4, 5, 6"). To establish *your* exhalation time, count during a comfortable exhalation. Don't force air out to the point of discomfort.

Pursed lip breathing is a basic technique used with all other breathing exercises and physical activities. Pursed lip breathing should be used whenever you do work or if your breathing becomes work. Remember to "whistle when you work." When you become short of breath, pursed lip breathing should be practiced along with diaphragmatic breathing. Learn it first and learn it well.

Diaphragmatic Breathing

The diaphragmatic breathing exercise will reactivate and strengthen the diaphragm. Normally the diaphragm does about 80% of the work of breathing. In patients with COPD the diaphragm flattens and the upper chest muscles are often used and eventually take over. These muscles are less efficient and require more oxygen to do the diaphragm's job. To locate your diaphragm, place your flat hand on your abdomen just below your breastbone—then sniff. You will feel your diaphragm move.

EXERCISE 1 CORRECT BREATHING TECHNIQUES WITH FRONT EXPANSION

Assume a comfortable position as indicated in the picture.

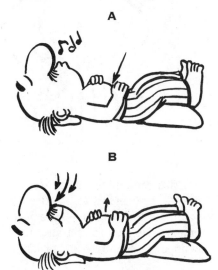

1. Place one hand in the center of your abdomen at the base of your breastbone—this hand will detect the movement of your diaphragm.

2. Place your other hand on your upper chest—this hand will detect any movement of your chest and accessory muscles.

3. Exhale slowly through pursed lips while pulling your abdominal muscles inward, squeezing them upward (Figure A).

4. Inhale slowly through your nose—your abdomen should expand downward and outward (Figure B). The hand over the diaphragm should feel the most movement.

5. Rest.

 EXERCISE 2 LOWER SIDE RIB BREATHING

Assume a comfortable sitting or standing position and good posture.

1. Place your hands on your sides at the base of your ribs.

2. Breathe out slowly through pursed lips, squeezing with the abdominal muscles. Your ribs and abdomen should move inward (Figure C).

3. Breathe in slowly through your nose and allow your ribs and abdomen to expand outward against your hands (Figure D).

4. Rest.

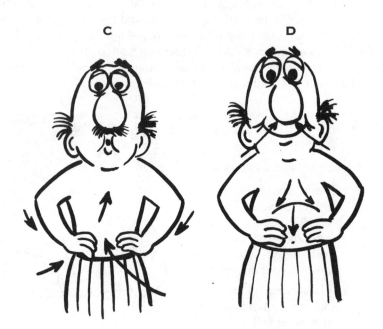

C   D

Practice combining these exercises after you have mastered them.

It is necessary to practice often in order to strengthen and coordinate your muscles. Set aside several (three to five) times throughout the day to practice. Be sure to rest after five deep breaths, or you may become lightheaded. Concentrate on making each breath slow and deep. Pursed lip breathing should always be used first to clear out the stale air when practicing *correct breathing*.

Diaphragmatic breathing can become your normal breathing pattern if practiced faithfully; this will result in less shortness of breath. Diaphragmatic and pursed lip breathing should be used during exercise and during strenuous activities, as well as during episodes of shortness of breath. Master these techniques before going on to other exercises.

Controlled Coughing Technique

Coughing is the natural way of removing foreign substances from the airways and lungs. Patients with chronic lung disease often produce an excess of mucus. Excess mucus must be removed to maintain open airways and allow you to move air in and out of your lungs effectively. If the excess mucus is not removed, shortness of breath can worsen. Retained mucus can also contribute to the risk of infection. In addition, the mucus irritates nerve endings in the tracheobronchial tree and can cause frequent, involuntary coughing, resulting in fatigue. To conserve energy and oxygen, practice and master the method of controlled coughing.

Step 1   At the end of a comfortable pursed lip exhalation, take a slow deep breath, using diaphragmatic breathing. Building up a volume of air behind the mucus will help to propel it toward the mouth.

Step 2   Hold the deep breath for several seconds.

Step 3   Cough twice with your mouth slightly open. The first cough loosens the mucus and the second cough moves it.

Step 4   Pause.

Step 5   Inhale by sniffing gently, or pant until you can take in another slow diaphragmatic breath. Taking in a big breath after coughing may cause you to cough again or may draw the mucus back into the lungs.

Step 6   Rest.

Using your inhaled medications and taking a drink of water before coughing can be helpful. Coughing is easier when you are in a sitting position with your head slightly forward. Controlled, effective coughing should make a hollow sound.

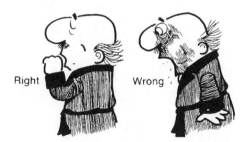

Right   Wrong

COUGHING STEPS IN BRIEF

1. Deep breathe.
2. Hold your breath.

3. Cough twice.

4. Pause.

5. Inhale by sniffing gently.

6. Rest.

If you need to cough again, repeat the procedure step by step. Control your cough; don't let it control *you*.

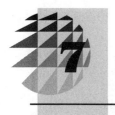

Day In, Day Out: Your Daily Activities

The use of proper breathing techniques while going about your daily routine will enable you to do more with less shortness of breath. Pace your work and activities with a comfortable breathing pattern. Remember to whistle when you work, doing the most exertion while you exhale. Another hint will help you work with your body's natural movements: **inhale as you expand your chest, and exhale when you compress your chest and/or abdomen.** Pace your work to your capacity and always maintain a controlled breathing pattern. If you feel like taking a couple of breaths between the work, do so—then continue as described. It is not necessary to work on every exhalation.

RULES:

1. Begin all exercises and work with correct breathing techniques (CBT) and doing a pursed lip exhalation to clear stale air from the lungs.
2. Take a deep breath by using your diaphragm before doing any work (especially something strenuous).
3. Exhale during the exertion part of the work. The only exception is to inhale when expanding the chest and exhale when compressing the chest or abdomen.
4. Breathe out at least twice as long as you breathe in (e.g., inhale to the count of 2, exhale to the count of 4).
5. If your oxygen prescription includes use with exertion, it includes everyday activities like showering, grooming, and moving about, as well as exercise.

STANDING UP FROM A CHAIR

- Do a correct breathing technique cycle to cleanse your lungs.
- Take a deep breath by using your diaphragm.
- While breathing out through pursed lips, move forward on the chair, then rise to your feet.

GOING UP A FLIGHT OF STAIRS OR WALKING UP A HILL

- Do a correct breathing cycle to cleanse your lungs.
- Before you start to climb, take a deep breath by using your diaphragm. While exhaling through pursed lips, climb two or three stairs or take two or three steps up the incline.
- Stop and rest while breathing in with your diaphragm again.
- If you feel short of breath at this point, rest for a while, taking as many breaths as needed to feel comfortable again. When you are ready, continue in the manner just described.

BENDING

To tie shoes, put on socks, or pick up fallen treasures requires compressing the abdomen against the diaphragm and chest. Work **with** your body; **exhale through pursed lips whenever you bend and compress the abdomen.**

LIFTING LOADS

Do CBT before beginning to do work. Before lifting, straighten the spine by doing a pelvic tilt (described in detail in Chapter 11) to reduce low back stress. Take a deep breath by using your diaphragm. Bend at the knees and hips, not at the waist. Exhale through pursed lips; when lifting, hold the load close to your body and place the load where you wish.

Many people with chronic lung disease regard all arm movements, especially movements from the shoulders, as difficult and tiresome. The following examples show how to coordinate proper breathing with these movements. Remember to inhale as you expand your chest and exhale through pursed lips when you compress your chest or diaphragm.

RAISING THE ARMS TO DO WORK OR REACH

Do CBT to cleanse the lungs before beginning work. Take a deep breath using your diaphragm, while lifting your arms to shoulder level and expanding your chest, reaching for the intended goal. Exhale as you retrieve the object that you reached for and lower your arms.

PUSHING A BROOM, VACUUM CLEANER, OR LAWN MOWER

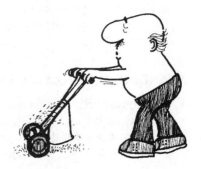

Do CBT to cleanse the lungs before beginning work. Take a deep breath by using your diaphragm before you start to push anything. Push objects while retaining straight posture and while exhaling with pursed lips. Stop and rest while inhaling, using your diaphragm. Continue coordinating breathing with pushing objects to do work.

SHAVING AND COMBING HAIR

Do a CBT to cleanse your lungs before beginning work. Take a deep breath, using your diaphragm, when you lift your arms and expand your chest. While exhaling, shave or comb two or three strokes. Lower your arms and rest before you run out of air. Your arms should be back in a resting position at the end of that comfortable exhalation. Do a CBT if necessary between activities. Remember that you need not work during each exhalation.

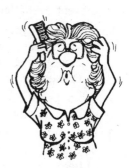

Some Additional Examples of when You Might Use this Breathing Technique

Household Tasks

Bedmaking
Window washing
Mopping
Moving furniture
Meal preparation/clean up

Exercises

Breathing exercises
Walking
Bicycle riding
Swimming
Body improvement exercises
Bronchial drainage
Relaxation exercises

Garden Work

Digging/planting
Raking leaves
Weeding

Hobbies

Golfing
Bowling
Swimming
Crafts

Personal Hygiene

Dressing
Brushing teeth
Showering

Some Examples of Energy Saving Techniques

Saving your energy can be important in order to complete your necessary daily chores. Often this can be accomplished by slight changes in the way you prioritize or perform these tasks.

1. Plan your daily chores in advance so that you won't feel rushed or have to push beyond your limitations.

2. Decide which jobs are absolutely necessary and which are desirable to make your home comfortable and attractive.

3. Adopt a cooperative work-sharing attitude within your family. Assign tasks and responsibilities.

4. Pace all work to your own breathing comfort and speed.

5. Distribute tedious tasks throughout the week.

6. Do the tasks requiring the most exertion when you have the most energy. For example, if mornings are difficult, take your shower and set the breakfast table the evening before.

7. Alternate easy and difficult activities, and take rest periods between to prevent overfatigue.

8. Save 50% of your energy: sit down to do your work. Use a stool at the kitchen counter, at the work bench, or in the shower.

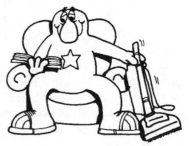

9. Drain dishes; let them air dry instead of towel drying.

10. Prepare food for two or more meals at one cooking session. Refrigerate or freeze individual size meals for another time.

11. Minimize clutter in storage areas, cupboards, closets, wardrobes, and tool sheds so that you can easily find and reach what you need.

12. Avoid ironing clothes by using easy care, no-iron fabrics.

13. Straighten up rooms as you go along. A good rule is "never leave a room empty-handed."

14. Vacuuming may leave fine dust in the air. Lightly misting the bag will reduce the number of escaping particles. To minimize breathing these particles in, try using a moist handkerchief in front of your mouth and nose while vacuuming; open windows and let the room air out for at least an hour. Use only disposable vacuum bags and change them often.

15. When making your bed, start at the head and progress down one side toward and across the foot, tucking in and smoothing as you go. Then proceed up the other side. Casters make moving the bed easier. It is more convenient if only the head of the bed is against the wall. Use an electric blanket. They are light weight, easy to lift, and don't weigh heavily on your body at night.

SOME TIPS FOR DAILY SELF-CARE

Your hygiene and grooming can be some of the more strenuous and exerting activities you have to do in a day. Sit while washing, showering, dressing, and grooming to conserve 50% of your energy!

1. A short, easy-to-maintain haircut requires less work, energy, and breath.

2. Try an electric toothbrush if brushing is a chore.

3. If you feel short of breath under an overhead shower or when splashing water on your face, use a washcloth, and install a hand shower to control the direction and force of the water flow.

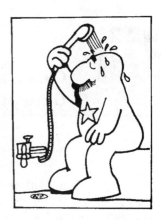

4. If steam in the shower bothers you, try turning on the cold water first and then slowly adding the hot. Leave the door ajar or use an exhaust fan to reduce steam.

5. Grab bars and no-slip strips in the tub or shower will help you keep your balance.

6. Avoid scented soaps, colognes, and other grooming products if you find they bother your breathing.

7. Keep your movements small and close to your body. You need not reach the ceiling to wash under your arm. To scrub your back, use a folded towel with handles at each end and a brush or loofah sponge attached in the middle; this is easy to pull diagonally back and forth across your back.

8. Try wrapping yourself in a terry cloth robe. Its absorbent qualities will dry you automatically. Rubbing yourself dry after a bath can be very tiring.

9. Be sure to use your oxygen in the shower or bath if it has been prescribed for use with activity. The portable tank with extra-long tubing can be set just outside the shower or tub.

10. Keep bathroom windows and doors open as much as possible to increase air flow and decrease steam buildup. Consider using a fan. The air does not necessarily have to be fresh for you to breathe comfortably, as long as it circulates.

Remember to coordinate your breathing techniques with all of these activities:

1. Use the diaphragm and relax the accessory muscles when you inhale.

2. Use pursed lips and squeeze with the abdominal muscles and diaphragm while you exhale. Exhale at least twice as long as you inhale.

3. Begin all activities with correct breathing techniques (CBT), starting with an exhalation to cleanse the lungs of trapped, stale air.

4. Inhale when expanding the chest and lungs.

5. Exhale when compressing the chest and/or abdomen.

8 Cleaning Out Your Tubes: Bronchial Drainage

Many people with chronic lung disease have secretions in their bronchial tubes that not only make it more difficult to breathe but also may interfere with getting oxygen into the blood. These secretions are also a perfect place for bacteria to grow and multiply and cause a major lung infection. By draining these secretions, you will be able to breathe more easily, prevent infections, and generally feel better.

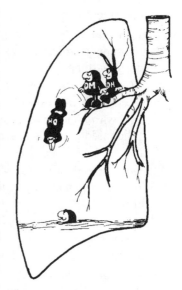

Secretions tend to pool in the bottom of your lungs because you spend most of your time in the upright position. To get secretions to a point where you can cough them up more easily, you must tilt your chest so that, with the assistance of gravity, the bronchial tubes of the lower lung areas can drain. This is called bronchial drainage.

You should learn techniques of bronchial drainage from a therapist or nurse only when ordered by your doctor. If you have high blood pressure or a history of strokes, do not perform bronchial drainage without discussing it with your doctor. Some basic points, the steps to follow, and pictures of bronchial drainage positions will help you to remember what you have learned.

BASIC POINTS

- Bronchial drainage is best done first thing in the morning (1 hour before breakfast) and in the evening (at least 1 hour before bedtime).
- Do bronchial drainage at least once or twice daily. Increase the number of treatments to three or four if your secretions change color or increase in amount or when you have a cold.
- When you feel like doing your bronchial drainage the least, you probably need it the most.

- If you use supplemental oxygen, be sure to use it while doing your bronchial drainage.
- It is most important to tilt the chest area 10 to 20 degrees below the horizontal level. This can be accomplished by using one of the following suggested methods:

> A slant board
> Couch pillows placed on the floor
> Firm pillows propped under your hips in bed

Steps to Follow for Effective Bronchial Drainage

STEP 1 *Conditioning of airways and secretions*

> Take prescribed medications to dilate your airways before you begin bronchial drainage. Oral bronchodilator medicine should ideally be taken at least 30 minutes beforehand. Inhaled bronchodilator medicines should be taken at least 10 minutes before doing bronchial drainage.
>
> Drink at least 1½ quarts of liquid daily. Adequate fluid intake is mandatory to keep mucus thin.

STEP 2 *Good inflation of the lungs*

> Breathing exercises are extremely important. Diaphragmatic and pursed lip breathing should be done throughout the bronchial drainage period. They help widen your airways so secretions can be drained more easily.

STEP 3 *Use of gravity, percussion, and vibration*

> The use of gravity is the most important aspect of draining secretions. The positions in the figures show gravity drainage positions. Stay in each position (1 through 4) for 5 to 15 minutes.

1. Both lower lobes

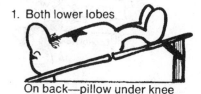

On back—pillow under knee

3. Right lower lobe

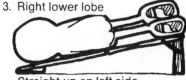

Straight up on left side

2. Left lower lobe

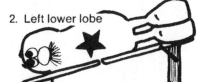

Straight up on right side

4. Both lower lobes

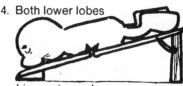

Lie on stomach

Percussion and vibration are additional methods of loosening secretions. Percussion may be prescribed for at least 1 minute in each position. Percussion, or clapping with a cupped hand on the chest wall, helps to move secretions into larger airways. Percussion should be done only on the rib cage and not over the spinal column, breastbone, or soft tissues.

Vibration is the other means of moving secretions. Your rib cage may be vibrated by another person or by a mechanical device. Vibration should follow percussion and is done for an additional minute only when you are exhaling.

Your skin should be covered with clothing or a towel during percussion and vibration. Your doctor or therapist should instruct you in these procedures.

If additional positions are needed, your doctor, therapist, or nurse will prescribe them.

STEP 4 *Controlled coughing*

Cough after each position, but only if you feel you need to and are sitting upright. Use the controlled coughing technique. Rest after coughing.

Precautions

If you have high blood pressure or a heart problem, be sure to check with your doctor before doing bronchial drainage. If you are taking steroids or have osteoporosis (brittle bones), check with your doctor before doing percussion or vibration on your chest.

REMEMBER THESE FOUR KEY STEPS:

1. Condition airways and secretions.
2. Inflate lungs.
3. Use gravity drainage.
4. Cough after each position.

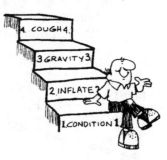

9   The Joy of Exercise

FIRST THINGS FIRST

Good physical condition is an objective that everyone should seek; the person with chronic lung disease is no exception. Individuals with chronic lung disease frequently avoid physical activity because of the limitations imposed by shortness of breath. In addition, friends, family, or physicians may have encouraged them not to exert themselves, assuming that to do so might cause "harmful effects." After years of study, we now know this is not true. *Inactivity* is an *enemy* working against you! Sitting 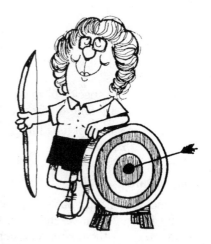 or lying around deconditions the body and makes all of your muscles less strong and less efficient. This in turn makes doing even the simplest daily activities more difficult, in terms of both energy and breathing. This deconditioning effect can be reversed by a regular exercise program.

The three major systems involved in exercise are the skeletal muscles, specialized heart muscles, and respiratory muscles. With progressive exercise of any kind, the fibers of the muscles involved become stronger and more resistant to fatigue. Also, with practice and training, you learn to perform tasks more efficiently; that is, you need less oxygen for the same amount of work. Thus you may have more "energy" to accomplish the tasks you perform each day, and you may do these tasks with less shortness of breath.

The reconditioning of muscles should be undertaken with great care, since suddenly starting to exercise may be useless at best and hazardous at worst. The proper way to approach improving your physical condition depends on two fundamentals:

1. Choosing appropriate goals
2. Your overall health at the time you start a physical conditioning program

In goal-setting, the athlete is limited by his or her natural abilities, body build, and motivation. A 4-foot 10-inch tall athlete should not aim at being a star professional basketball player. The person with chronic lung disease is subject to these same limitations in goal-setting, plus an additional one: the status of his or her lung function. Careful evaluation of the type and extent of your lung function abnormalities is es-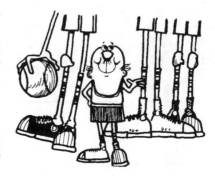 sential before establishing a physical conditioning program. Such evaluation is required for two reasons:

1. Certain specific physical conditioning techniques can help the person with lung disease to improve lung function itself.
2. The status of lung function must be known to establish safe limits of exercise.

Play It Safe

You should consult your physician before beginning an exercise program. You can then work together in choosing the type of exercise that is most useful and best fits in with your life-style.

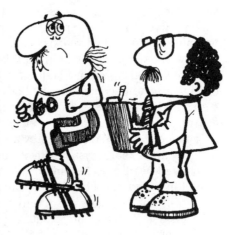

Each part of your physical conditioning program should be checked for safety before you attempt it. For example, walking too far, too quickly may put excessive strain on your lungs or heart. Or certain physical activities may cause your blood oxygen level to fall too low, requiring supplemental oxygen during exercise. Do not attempt to construct your own program. Your doctor and other health care professionals will guide you within safe limits. These limits can be established only by appropriate testing. The program must then be tailored to your specific lung, heart, and other limitations. There are no simple guidelines that you can establish. For instance, becoming short of breath during a given exercise does not mean that you are overdoing it and have to stop. If it did, most athletes would stop in the middle of a race, a tennis match, or a football game. Remember to use pursed lip and diaphragmatic breathing. If you have COPD, try to exhale twice as long as you inhale. Even fatigue or aching muscles do not necessarily mean you are overdoing it. It may be necessary to experience such discomforts to improve your condition. Let your physician set the limits based on detailed knowledge of your condition.

Components of an Exercise Program

Each exercise session should include three phases:

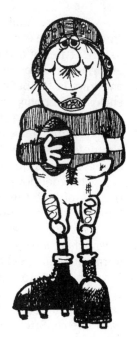

1. A warm-up
2. An aerobic activity (exercise that requires oxygen, uses your large muscle groups and can be sustained for a period of time such as walking, running, bicycling, or swimming)
3. A cool-down

The warm-up phase of your exercise program should precede stretching and aerobic exercise and lasts 5 to 10 minutes. The purpose of the warm-up is to prepare the body for the greater demands of exercise by promoting body awareness and to increase blood flow and oxygen to the muscles. This increase in your internal temperature increases muscle elasticity, thereby increasing flexibility of tendons and ligaments and decreasing the potential risk of injury. Beginning exercise too suddenly may put a strain on your heart or make your lung function worse, thereby increasing shortness of breath. Bronchodilating inhalers should be nearby and used before beginning exercise. Movements used in the warm-up should specifically prepare the body for movements used during the exercise component. If you are going to walk, you can do chair exercises that simulate walking, or walk at a slower pace.

The kind of exercise that will benefit you most depends on what you want to do. Exercise training is rather specific: weight-lifting, swimming, bicycling, running, dancing, jumping, calisthenics, and so on, all "train" different muscles. Most people with chronic lung disease want to increase their ability to walk in terms of duration and intensity. Walking is one of the best forms of exercise for three reasons:

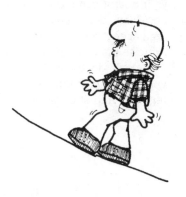

1. It uses many body muscles, including the heart and diaphragm
2. It requires no special equipment or skill
3. It can be measured easily (speed, distance)

Therefore, walking is the usual starting point for most people with chronic lung disease. From this starting point you may want to branch out to other types of aerobic exercise. Attention should be paid to extremes in environmental conditions such as air pollution, pollen counts, and highs and lows in temperature. If necessary, walk inside your home or go to an enclosed shopping mall.

Duration of the aerobic phase is related to your functional capacity and may vary from a few minutes to an hour. The *frequency* may vary from three 5-minute sessions or two 15-minute sessions daily to one 30-minute session every day or every other day.

The cool-down after exercise lowers your heart rate, helps prevent pooling of blood in the lower extremities, and reduces muscle soreness. Similar to the warm-up, the cool-down should last 5 to 10 minutes.

Stretching may be used in combination with the warm-up or cool-down when your internal temperature is increased and your muscles are warm. Stretching enhances flexibility. Flexibility is important to prevent injury and to improve physical performance. A stretch should be performed slowly with control and held, *without bouncing*. Muscles involved in the exercise you plan to perform or have already performed should be the focus of each stretch. Stretching also plays an integral part in stress reduction and muscle relaxation (see Chapter 10).

Your Job

Whatever the exercise program designed for you, you will be responsible for mastering it. You will find that you may have to push yourself to establish a regular routine. Being short of breath creates a temptation to remain inactive, especially on the days when the shortness of breath may seem worse. When planning a safe exercise schedule, remember to start slowly. Plan a progressive walking program, beginning with short distances and a slow pace. You may gradually increase the duration of your walks as your strength and endurance increase. Keep a careful record of your exercise sessions, for example, how long you walked, how fast you walked, your pulse rate before and after, and how you tolerated the exercise. Then you and your doctor can monitor your progress and adjust your exercise routine as necessary. Setting aside a specific time to exercise may help to establish a regular regimen. Finding a companion to exercise *with* you can make your exercise program more enjoyable and help with motivation.

Your doctor and other health professionals can guide you. But it is your job to pick up the ball and carry it through by following the program regularly and sticking with it. Let's go!

10 Letting Go: Relaxation Techniques

WHY TALK ABOUT RELAXATION?

When you are physically and emotionally relaxed, you avoid excessive oxygen consumption caused by tension of overworked muscles. Relaxation also decreases other undesirable manifestations of stress such as mental irritability and anxiety that might induce bronchospasm, increased shortness of breath, and fatigue. By using some of the suggested relaxation methods outlined in the following sections, you can relieve the tension that increases your respiratory difficulties. Complete muscular relaxation is also important to gain maximal benefits from all other exercises.

The key to relaxation is, above all, breathing control. When you can master diaphragmatic breathing, relaxation of the accessory muscles, and prolonged exhalation with pursed lips at times of stress, you have achieved a major victory in the battle against panic. At such times you should also remember positioning, which can be either standing or sitting, but always leaning forward with your arms supported.

To practice this first progressive relaxation technique, lie down on a comfortable surface and place one pillow under your head and one under your knees. Having quiet, peaceful surroundings is helpful. The principle that applies here is that maximal relaxation follows maximal contraction. Always tighten and relax the muscles gradually.

Head and Neck

1. Pull your chin down toward your chest as tightly as possible and push the back of your head into the pillow, then let go.

2. Turn your head from side to side in a relaxed manner.

3. Let it stop when it comes to a comfortable position.

Shoulders

1. Shrug your shoulders and tighten the shoulder muscles as much as possible.

2. Let go.

59

Arms

1. Do one hand and one arm at a time.

2. Bend your elbow and make a fist out of your hand. Tighten as much as possible, then let go.

3. Straighten your arm and fingers. Tighten as much as possible, then let go.

Legs

1. Do one leg at a time.

2. Straighten your leg and point your toes; tighten as much as possible, then let go.

3. Pull your toes toward your nose and push your heel and back of your leg into the bed.

4. Tighten as much as possible, then let go.

Back

1. Arch your back up in that slow, easy way a cat does.

2. Do not lift your hips while arching. Tighten as much as possible, then let go.

Face

1. Tighten (scrinch) all of your face muscles.

2. Hold, then let go.

Eyes

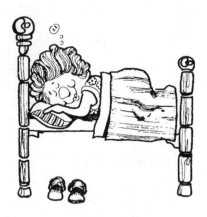

1. Try to focus your eyes on something. Watch it and slowly let your eyelids grow heavy.

2. Open your eyes and let them close gradually until they feel comfortable closed. Sweet dreams!

OTHER RELAXATION TECHNIQUES

Another way to control your tension is to create in your mind a mental picture of something that gives you a good and comfortable feeling. This may be a scene, real or imagined: a landscape with rolling hills, green grass, and trees with their leaves gently moving in the wind; or the beach; a poolside; or your mother's kitchen. Try to make your mental picture detailed.

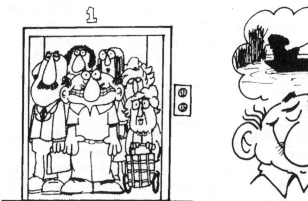 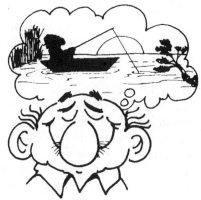

Each time you find yourself in a difficult situation that you cannot immediately leave (for example, a crowded elevator), use the visual image you have created as a mental escape. This will help keep your anxiety and shortness of breath under control until you can physically remove yourself from that situation.

"Mind-over-matter" relaxation techniques are another way to help increase your mind's awareness and control over your body. There are many different ways to do this type of "self-hypnosis." You can simply concentrate on a certain part of your body; for instance, concentrate on your right hand and envision that it is becoming very limp, soft, heavy, or light. Any of these sensations will induce relaxation. Sometimes during a stressful or anxiety-provoking event, blood will rush to the center of the body, leaving the limbs cool and moist. Thinking of your hands and feet as "getting warm" is very effective, since relaxation will occur when the temperature increases. Try it first with one hand and, when you have succeeded in warming it, proceed up the arm, to the shoulder, then to the other hand, and so on until you have finally "told" your whole body to relax and it has obeyed you.

Another useful relaxation technique is one most frequently used in different types of meditation. Concentrate on one word and repeat it over and over to yourself (such as the word "free"). Repeat the word each time you breathe out. Do not let yourself get distracted by intruding thoughts; ignore them and return to repeating your word. Don't be concerned about how deep a relaxation level you are reaching. When trying these different modes of relaxation exercises, become passive and allow relaxation to come about at its own pace.

Sleep eradicates the effects of daily fatigue. Many people with chronic lung disease, however, have trouble sleeping, sometimes because of their medications. The events of modern life, in addition, frequently overload human faculties, causing exhaustion that may not be corrected by sleep. Meditation is thought to produce an extraordinarily deep rest and a stress release much more complete than sleep. It is particularly suited for gradual removal of long-accumulated stress. This may be one relaxation method you will want to investigate further. Meditation can be used in conjunction with the progressive relaxation technique first mentioned. You start by relaxing your muscles, then you meditate.

Other modes of relaxation can include learning to give yourself a massage or having someone else give you one, especially on the neck and shoulder muscles. The vibrator you use for bronchial drainage can be very useful for this purpose also (see Chapter 8). Biofeedback is another way to learn to relax and explore your own ability to control tension and shortness of breath. You might have already found your own way to relax, be it soft music, yoga, or a bubble bath. There are many simple techniques worth trying. If they work for you, use them!

Making Your Body Work Better

BODY IMPROVEMENT EXERCISES

The techniques described here will not help the lungs themselves but will improve your entire physical condition. These body improvement exercises will increase the efficiency of your muscles so that they require less fuel (oxygen) during exertion.

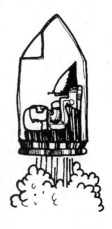

Before starting these exercises, you want to be sure that your lungs are as "clean" as possible. So if you have excess mucus, you should clear your lungs of mucus by the techniques already described before beginning these exercises. If you are tense, total body relaxation techniques should be followed before exercise. And if pursed lip breathing or diaphragmatic breathing has been prescribed for you, you should use these methods during exercise.

In other words, you should have "all systems go" before "blasting off" into body improvement exercises. This is like the athlete who warms up before a big event. Once you are warmed up, you can get started!

Each of these exercises may be performed two to ten times daily after first checking with your physician or therapist regarding your specific physical limitations (see Chapter 9). Start the exercise program by doing just a couple of repetitions of each exercise. Increase the repetitions gradually.

WARM UP EXERCISES TO RELAX SHOULDER AND NECK MUSCLES

The shoulder and neck muscles are considered accessory breathing muscles and are not normally involved in the work of quiet breathing. Some individuals with chronic lung disease tend to breathe shallowly, using upper chest muscles because of decreased mobility of the rib cage and flattening of the diaphragm. To breathe properly, you must relax your shoulder and neck muscles. The following exercises can be done any time during the day when you feel tension in the shoulder and neck area. They should also be done between the other exercises in your body improvement program.

EXERCISE: SHOULDER SHRUGGING

1. Stand or sit with feet slightly apart and arms relaxed.
2. Shrug your shoulders and tighten the muscles as much as possible.
3. Relax and rest.
4. Repeat up to ten times.

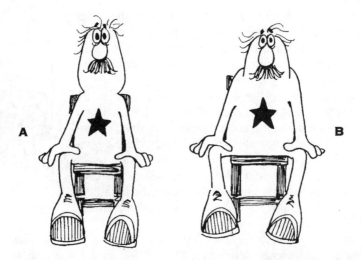

EXERCISE: ELBOW CIRCLING

1. Sit or stand with hands on shoulders.
2. Circle the elbows forward, up, back, and downward. Do two to ten circles.
3. Relax muscles.

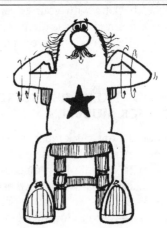

EXERCISE: HEAD CIRCLING

1. Roll your head slowly from side to side in a forward semicircle.
2. Repeat a couple of times.
3. Do *not* arch your neck by rolling your head back.

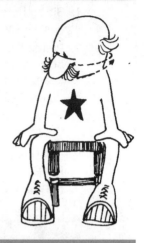

EXERCISE: CIRCLING OF SHOULDERS WITH HANGING ARMS

1. Sit or stand with arms relaxed.
2. Circle your left shoulder up and back.
3. Repeat up to ten times.
4. Repeat on the right side.
5. Finally circle both shoulders together.
6. Repeat up to ten times.
7. Repeat the exercise in opposite direction.

A

B

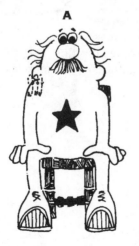
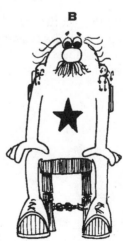

EXERCISE: OVER-THE-HEAD SHOULDER STRETCH

1. Sit and press your lower back firmly against the back of the chair.

2. Pretend you are holding a stick. Keep both arms outstretched three feet apart. Do not lock your elbows.

3. Slowly raise your extended arms above your head to the point where the top of your shoulders feels tight.

4. Hold the position at the tightest place for 5 to 10 seconds.

5. Return to starting position and relax.

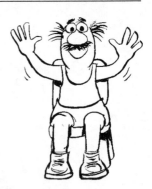

EXERCISE: UNDERNEATH SHOULDER STRETCH

1. Sit and bend your head and chest forward slightly.

2. Reach your arms behind your back, clasp your hands together, and lift slowly.

3. Hold the position at the point where the muscles feel the tightest for 5 to 10 seconds.

4. Return to starting position and re-lax.

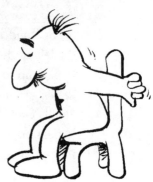

COMMENTS: Do the last two stretching exercises once each. Try to gradually increase the holding time of the stretched position up to the point where you feel a release of the tightness in the muscles.

WARM UP EXERCISES TO INCREASE MOBILITY OF THE RIB CAGE

Some individuals with chronic lung disease develop stiff rib cages, especially the lower ribs. If this is a problem, the following group of exercises will help to increase the mobility of the rib cage. This enables the lower lung areas to expand more fully.

EXERCISE: FORWARD BENDING

1. Sit in a straight-back chair, feet flat on the floor and slightly apart, shoulders relaxed, arms comfortable at the sides (Figure A).

2. While exhaling, drop your head to your chest and slowly roll your body forward, toward your knees, keeping your back rounded (not straight) (Figures B and C).

3. While inhaling, return to the upright position slowly by pushing first your lower, then middle, then upper back against the chair.

4. Relax, and repeat up to ten times.

A

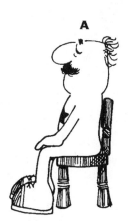

B

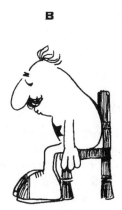

C

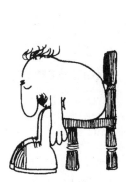

EXERCISE: SIDE BENDING

1. Sit up straight with feet apart.
2. While exhaling slowly, bend your head and shoulders to the left while exhaling (Figure A).
3. Return to starting position while inhaling and rest.
4. Repeat on the other side (Figure B).
5. Repeat up to ten times on both sides.

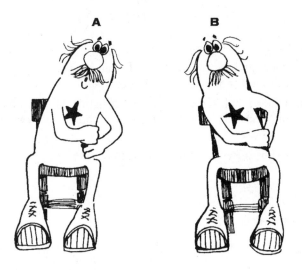

EXERCISES TO IMPROVE ARM PERFORMANCE

Since arm movement can be very strenuous for individuals with chronic lung disease, it is important to maintain muscle strength and endurance with simple arm exercises. Work both arms simultaneously, maintaining the muscle tension as you do each exercise. Do not suddenly relax or drop the arms. Coordinate lifts with breathing, developing a rhythmic pattern of inhaling in conjunction with the positive (expanding the chest) movements and exhaling with the negative (compressing the chest) movements of the exercise.

Initially perform one set of ten repetitions of each arm exercise. Rest one minute between each set. As your strength and endurance improve, proceed to two sets of ten repetitions of each exercise, using the same weight. Finally, proceed to three sets. Complete the various sets of each exercise consecutively. When you can comfortably do three sets of ten lifts of all the arm exercises, you may increase your weights by one pound.

After a weight increase, begin with one set of ten lifts of each exercise, gradually progressing toward three sets of ten lifts of each exercise. Do your weight lifting exercise every other day. Do not use weights heavier than four pounds for men and three pounds for women.

During the arm exercises performed in a chair, sit with your hip and knee joints at 90-degree angles with your feet flat on the floor. Press your lower back firmly against the back of the chair during arm activity. Do not allow an increase in the curvature of your lower back. Lift your arms initially only as far as you can without arching your back. Do not lock your elbows during weight lifting. If pain or other unusual symptoms arise during arm exercise, *stop* the painful motion and *do not repeat*. Coordinate correct breathing techniques with the motion.

 EXERCISE: DIAGONAL ARM RAISES

1. Sit in a straight back chair with your feet slightly apart and your arms crossed in your lap.

2. While inhaling, lift your arms upward and out in a straight diagonal.

3. On exhalation, reverse the motion and return to the starting position.

4. Repeat up to ten times.

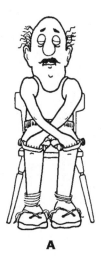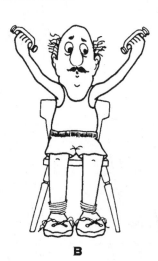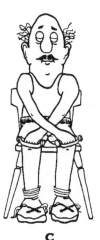

A   **B**   **C**

EXERCISE: SIDEWARD ARM RAISES

1. Sit in a straight back chair with feet slightly apart and arms down at your sides.
2. While inhaling, lift your arms out and up until they are vertical above your head.
3. On exhalation, reverse the motion and return to the starting position.
4. Repeat up to ten times.

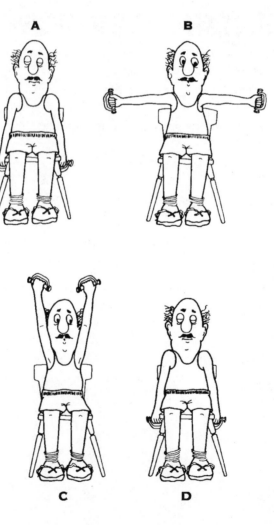

EXERCISE: SIDE FORWARD ARM RAISES

1. Sit in a straight back chair with feet slightly apart and arms down at your sides.
2. While inhaling, lift your arms out and up to horizontal, then forward until your hands meet in front of your body.
3. On exhalation, reverse the motion and return to the starting position.
4. Repeat up to ten times.

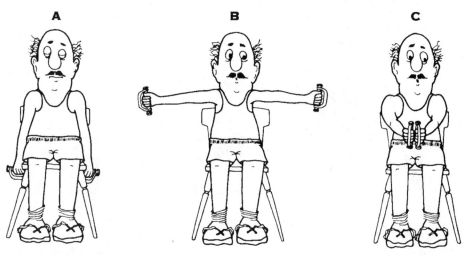

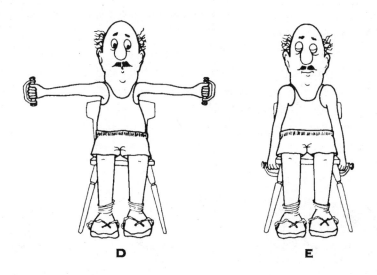

EXERCISE: STRAIGHT ARM RAISES BACKWARD AND FORWARD

1. Lie on your back with knees bent, feet flat on the floor, arms at sides, and weights in hands.
2. Keep the small of your back pressed against the floor.
3. While inhaling, lift straight arms up and back as far as you can without feeling movement in your back.
4. On exhalation, reverse the movement by bringing straight arms forward and down again by your sides.
5. Repeat up to ten times, then rest.

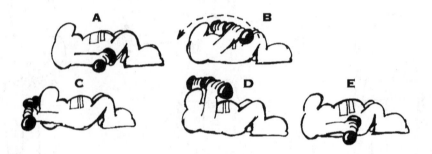

EXERCISE: ELBOW BENDS WITH ARMS UP

1. Lie on your back with knees bent, feet flat on the floor, arms at sides, and weights in hands.
2. While inhaling, bend your elbows.
3. Keep the small of your back pressed against the floor.
4. On the exhalation, straighten your arms up in the air and return to bent elbows.
5. Repeat up to ten times, then rest.

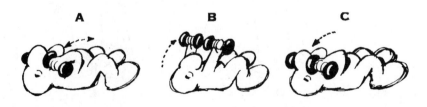

EXERCISE: STRAIGHT ARM RAISES INWARD AND OUTWARD

1. Lie with your arms at a 90-degree angle from your body (straight out from the sides).
2. Keep the small of your back pressed against the floor.
3. While inhaling, lift both arms straight up so your hands meet above your face.
4. Return to original position on exhalation.
5. Repeat up to ten times, then rest.

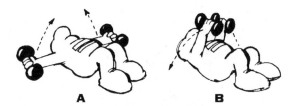

A   B

EXERCISES TO STRENGTHEN ABDOMINAL MUSCLES

Some people with chronic lung disease must work to get air *out* as well as *in*. Strong abdominal muscles can help push air out by compressing the rib cage and pulling the lower ribs downward. Through active exercise, the abdominal muscles can regain their elasticity and their capacity to relax. This aids diaphragmatic breathing, effective coughing, and muscular back support. These exercises must be done smoothly and slowly. You must contract your stomach muscles and press the small of your back against the floor while doing head, shoulder, and leg raises.

 EXERCISE: CONTRACTION OF ABDOMINAL MUSCLES WITH PELVIC TILT

1. Lie on your back with knees bent and feet flat on the floor. Place a pillow under your head (basic starting position, Figure A).
2. While exhaling, contract the abdominal muscles and roll your hips under so that your back is flat against the floor (Figure B).
3. Relax your muscles and rest.
4. Repeat up to ten times.
   NOTE: If you are unable to contract your abdominal muscles as described, start your exercise program with any of the following exercises until you gain awareness of the state of your abdominal muscles and how to use them.

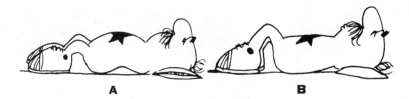

A   **B**

 ## EXERCISE: HEAD AND SHOULDER RAISING

1. Assume the basic starting position and cross your arms in front of your chest.
2. With your chin tucked in and while exhaling, raise your head and shoulders.
3. Return to the starting position while inhaling and then rest.
4. Repeat once.

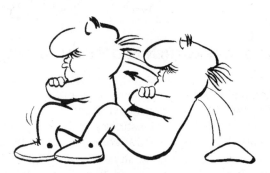

 ## EXERCISE: KNEE BENDING

1. Assume the basic starting position shown in Figure A.
2. While exhaling, bring the left knee toward your left shoulder and press the small of your back against the floor (Figure B).
3. Inhale while returning to the starting position and relax.
4. Repeat on the right side.
5. Repeat up to ten times on each side.

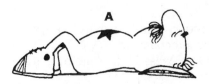 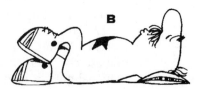

BODY MECHANICS

The joints and bones in your body are parts of a machine that will wear out if they are strained too much or incorrectly. Also, advancing age and long-term use of steroids may make bones brittle. Proper body mechanics are essential to make the whole of your body function effectively.

Yes

No

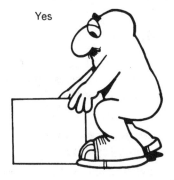
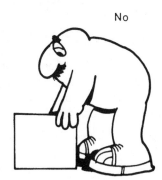

Pushing

- It is important that your motions be smooth and steady, never jerky or sudden.
- Do not lift, push, or pull when your back is twisted or bent. Use your feet to turn around, and lift by bending and straightening your knees. When you lift an object, it should be held as close to your body as possible.
- Avoid carrying heavy items in your arms; instead, use a rolling cart for groceries, laundry, and equipment.

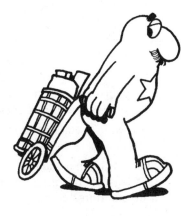

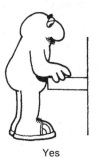
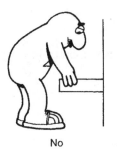
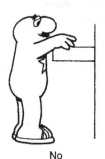

Yes   No   No

- Working surfaces should be of the proper height so you can avoid excessive back bending or having to lift your arms too high. Proper working area height is generally a couple of inches below your elbows, for both the standing and sitting positions.
- Never sit in a chair that's too low; have your back, feet, and arms well supported. You will generally feel more comfortable sitting erect or even leaning slightly forward.

REDEVELOPMENT OF GOOD POSTURE

Maintaining a well-balanced carriage is as essential to habitual good breathing as using your diaphragm and abdominal muscles and relaxing the shoulders, neck, and upper chest. The following basic points should be considered and practiced.

1. Stand with at least half the body weight carried forward over the front of the feet so that the toes are well pressed onto the ground.
2. Practice rocking forward until the heels have to come off the ground and then backward until the toes do, then settle between these two extremes. The weight should be at least evenly divided between the front of the foot and the heel. In most cases it is necessary to accentuate the forward-shifting of the weight.
3. Stand sideways in front of a long mirror and note the following:
   a. Is your head poking forward? Correct this by stretching upward and tucking your chin in while pressing your head backward.
   b. Is your seat sticking out? Tuck in the seat muscles and relax your shoulders and upper chest.
   c. Do your shoulders hunch forward? Bring your shoulder blades down and back.
4. When sitting in a chair, sit well back in the seat and support your legs on the floor (never dangle them). Support your arms on armrests or place them on your lap.

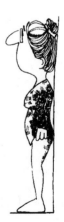

Practice Posture Work Against a Wall for About 5 Minutes at a Time

Assume the following position:

1. Place feet a few inches apart, a few inches away from the wall.
2. Hold head high.
3. Tuck chin in.
4. Relax shoulders.

5. Tuck hips under.

6. Slightly flex knees.

When you feel you can hold the position properly, try standing away from the wall in the proper postural position, and then attempt to walk in this position. You will notice that the trunk stays quite rigid but the legs (hips and knees) bend more when walking. Check to see if you have retained the proper position by backing up to the wall frequently during your walking practice. Do not stiffen up when trying to maintain a proper posture. Only by being relaxed can you benefit from this exercise.

12 You Are What You Eat

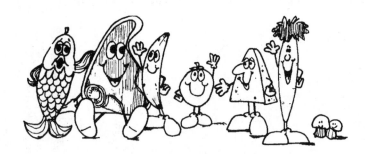

Eating is one of life's great pleasures. Food isn't just nourishment; it is associated with all types of significant events. What you eat may affect you emotionally and influence how well you function mentally. A healthful diet allows you to fight infection and disease and promotes a long and healthy life.

Nutrition and health are big business, and we are continually flooded with information. Newspapers, magazines, radio, and television have ads, articles, and commentaries about the subject. Some of the information comes from reliable sources; a lot of it does not. Nutrition is now "in." Whenever any health issue is popular, the public must be wary. People have to know *who* is saying *what*—and *why*. Daily there are stories that say "don't eat this" (it may kill you) or "do eat that" (it will cure whatever is wrong with you). One who reacts to all these stories can become confused at best and extremely anxious or sick at worst. Unfortunately, much of this information is incomplete or is based on either no scientific studies or a misinterpretation of the studies done. There is no question that good nutrition is important. There is also no question that there are well-meaning people who are convinced that eating sugar is "bad" or that taking large quantities of certain vitamins is "good." However, conviction, enthusiasm, and testimonials are no guarantee of scientific accuracy.

A sensible approach to nutrition begins with a basic understanding of how the body works and how it uses food to produce energy. The body and its digestive system are very smart. Most of the things you eat can be converted from one form to another by the body. It is very difficult to trick the digestive system. For example, the body requires sugar as an energy source. If you take none in, the body will make it out of other things you eat, or your "engine" will not run. Indeed, this ability of the digestive system to make the things it needs often saves us from ourselves when we go on strange fad diets. Given this marvelous, flexible manufacturing system, all we have to do to maintain good nutrition is to use common sense. Give the body an even break and it will serve you well. Therefore, the basic rule of good nutrition is a simple one: *eat everything in moderation*. Fad diets and fear about eating certain things are not warranted. Unless you have some kind of rare digestive disease, are truly allergic to some food (a very rare situation), have some kind of hereditary problem (again, quite rare), or have special medical problems, eating a regular, reasonably balanced diet is all you need to do. *Just avoid excesses*. Eating a gallon of ice cream a day does not make sense, nor does being terrified of eating a dish of ice cream. Salting foods until they are white is not moderation. There is no reason to challenge your body. Treat it reasonably. Eat things in moderation.

It certainly is a fact that with decreased physical activity, you need fewer calories to burn for energy; yet you still need protein, carbohydrates, fats, vitamins, and minerals. You can manage this balancing act by avoiding an excess of foods that provide mainly calories but few nutrients, such as sweets, fast foods, and packaged "goodies." Give some thought to your choices and select those foods that give you more of the nutrients you need.

An important goal for the individual with chronic lung disease is to maintain ideal body weight. This may be not the weight on the life insurance charts but the weight you felt best at and maintained through most of your adult life. Many of us gain extra weight in the midriff or stomach region. For the person with lung disease, this extra weight could mean increased shortness of breath because of the added pressure on the diaphragm. The diaphragm is the drum-like structure under the lungs that is responsible for much of the lungs' movement. Eating a large meal, consuming liquids during the meal, or eating foods that cause gas and distention may put pressure on the diaphragm, which causes difficult breathing. Being underweight can affect the ability to fight infection and fatigue. Discuss your dietary goals with your physician and dietician. They can provide information on weight maintenance for optimal health.

THE ESSENTIAL NUTRIENTS

There are six nutrients that are necessary for health:

Water

Water is responsible for approximately two thirds of your total weight. It not only helps to digest food and eliminate waste but, for individuals with lung disease, it also helps to keep mucus and secretions thin. Mucus that accumulates in the airways is a breeding ground for infection. If you are underweight, choose liquids high in calories such as milk shakes and fruit nectars. If you are overweight, water is always a good choice. The person with chronic lung disease should drink eight to ten glasses of fluid per day. When adding up your fluid intake, don't include beverages with alcohol or caffeine, because both cause you to lose fluid. You needn't worry about increased mucus from dairy products; there is no evidence that milk products produce mucus in lung tissue.

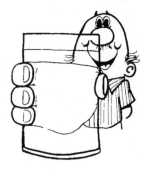

Protein

This group provides essential amino acids the body uses to repair and maintain tissue. Dairy products, fish, poultry, and meat are good choices. Choose the low-fat varieties and trim any visible fat. Beans and legumes are also good sources of protein when combined with whole grains. This combination provides a complete protein source that is low in fat and high in fiber.

Carbohydrates

Carbohydrates come in two categories: simple and complex. Simple carbohydrates are sugary type "treats," and complex carbohydrates include whole grains, breads, cereals, rice, and pasta. Consuming simple carbohydrates may cause an increase in carbon dioxide production, which may contribute to shortness of breath. Complex carbohydrates contain many vitamins and minerals and the fiber essential to good health. Make them your frequent choice and consume simple carbohydrates only on an occasional basis.

Fat

Fat contains "essential fatty acids," which must be supplied by the diet. It's easy to consume enough fat; however, some choices are better than others. The best choices are the monounsaturated fats that include canola, olive, and peanut oil. These fats are the least likely to raise blood cholesterol levels. Polyunsaturated fats are the next best choice. Saturated fats—the "hard fats" that include the marbling in beef, lard, tropical oils, butter, and margarine—are the least desirable. These have the greatest potential for increasing cholesterol levels.

Vitamins

Vitamins help to turn food into energy. Their functions vary widely and are essential to health.

Vitamin A is important for growth and vision and to fight infection. Beta-carotene, a pigment found in the plant kingdom, is converted to vitamin A in the body. Good sources of vitamin A or beta-carotene include liver, dark leafy greens, and any yellow-orange vegetables.

The B vitamins are important for nerve function, digestion, appetite, healthy skin, and converting carbohydrate to energy. Some good sources are whole-grain products, meat, poultry, fish, nuts, and dairy products.

Vitamin C is important, but the amount needed is still in question. Some excellent sources include oranges, grapefruits, strawberries, broccoli, cantaloupe, and potatoes. Eating at least five servings of fruits and vegetables per day assures a healthful intake of this vitamin.

Vitamin D is produced when the human body is exposed to sunlight. Most dairy products and dry cereals are fortified with vitamin D. Some other good sources include sardines, fresh salmon, canned tuna, and shrimp.

Vitamin E is also a controversial supplement. Like vitamins A and D, it is a fat-soluble vitamin and is stored in tissue. It's always a good idea to check with a dietician or physician before adding supplements to your diet. Good sources of vitamin E include vegetable oils, nuts, wheat germ, and legumes.

Minerals

Minerals help maintain vital body functions and help manufacture bones, blood, and teeth. Some medications taken by people with chronic lung disease can interfere with absorption of calcium. Calcium is especially important for women, who are at greater risk for osteoporosis. Dairy products provide the best sources of calcium. Check with your physician regarding your drug–nutrient interactions.

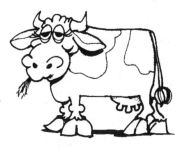

Vitamins and minerals are essential to good health and can easily be provided by a varied and balanced diet. Always be wary of supplement advertisements making unrealistic promises. Not only are supplements expensive—they can be dangerous.

Eating well is important to everyone, but the individual with chronic lung disease has special needs. Some potential nutritional problems and solutions are included in the following section.

GAS AND DISTENTION

Eating too much at one sitting or eating certain gas-producing foods can cause a "bloated" feeling, put pressure on the diaphragm, and make breathing difficult.

SOLUTION

1. Eat several small meals each day instead of three large ones. Drink fluids between meals rather than with meals. Eating small meals requires less energy expenditure.

2. Avoid gas-forming foods. Some common offenders include:

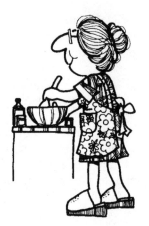

Apples	Carbonated drinks
Beans/legumes	Cauliflower
Beer	Onions
Broccoli	Radishes
Brussels sprouts	Sauerkraut
Cabbage	Sweets
Cantaloupe and other melons	Watermelon

3. Eat slowly and talk less during meals to avoid swallowing air. Don't exercise right before or right after eating. Consumption, digestion, and absorption of food require a significant amount of energy. Rest after eating.

LOSS OF MUSCLE MASS

Patients with lung disease often experience muscle wasting. A consistent exercise program helps preserve muscles and fight fatigue, and it can increase your energy level. Combine a healthful diet with exercise.

SOLUTION

1. Eat a varied and balanced diet. Emphasize fruits and vegetables (at least five servings per day).

2. Eat at least two servings of protein-rich foods per day. For example, two 3-ounce servings of meat, fish, or poultry. Beans/legumes and dairy products are also good choices.

3. Increase the protein and calorie content of your food by adding nonfat dry milk to sauces, gravies, cream dishes, casseroles, and desserts. You can add approximately ¼ cup of nonfat dry milk to many recipes without changing the flavor. Increase the protein and calorie content of milk by adding nonfat dry milk to regular milk; just mix well and chill.

LOSS OF APPETITE

Many people with chronic lung disease experience loss of appetite and weight loss. If you are underweight, it is important to keep track of your

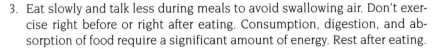

weight and strive for weight maintenance. Mucus production and some medications can also decrease appetite.

SOLUTION

1. Take medications with milk or meals unless otherwise advised.
2. Practice bronchial drainage an hour or two before meals.
3. Enjoy some fresh air and light exercise a short time before meals.
4. Prepare foods *you* enjoy that have enticing aromas. Vary your menus.
5. Celebrate your meals. Provide music, color, and outdoor locations for eating. Vary the colors and textures of your food.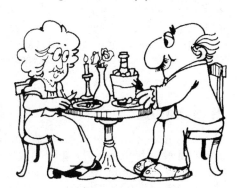
6. Share your meals with a friend or loved one.
7. Take advantage of community meal programs at churches and senior centers.

POTASSIUM DEPLETION

People with chronic lung disease may have low potassium levels. This may be due to diuretics (water pills), but usually the cause is unknown. Some signs of low potassium levels are weakness, tingling, numbness of the fingers, and leg cramps.

SOLUTION:

Consume foods high in potassium every day. Here are some examples:

Bananas	Mushrooms	Spinach
Broccoli	Oranges	Tomato products
Dried fruit	Peanuts	Winter squash
Dry skim milk	Potatoes	Yams

FLUID RETENTION

Foods high in salt (or sodium) often cause fluid retention. If you retain water or have high blood pressure, you may need to decrease the amount of salt in your diet. Salt is the most frequently used additive in the United States and is contained in almost all processed, canned, and fast foods. A dietician can provide helpful information on reducing sodium intake.

TIPS TO SAVE TIME AND ENERGY

Preparing meals can leave you fatigued, with little energy to enjoy your meal. Here are a few suggestions to make meal preparation easier:

1. Make one-dish meals (casseroles). These are easy to prepare and clean up.
2. Prepare large quantities and freeze in individual "packages" for future meals.
3. Pace yourself while cooking. Try not to rush when preparing a meal.
4. Use conveniences like a microwave or crock pot. These appliances can help you make more nutritious meals than you could using the conventional methods. Oven cooking requires less energy than stove top cooking.

IN CLOSING . . .

Check with your physician or dietician before taking supplements or trying a new dietary regimen. The goal is to eat healthful, nutritious food 80% to 90% of the time and to be aware of the foods you consume. There is an abundance of food available; with minimal planning and effort your meals can be a great source of pleasure while simultaneously providing strength, nourishment, and energy.

Good Luck!   Good Health!   Good Eating!

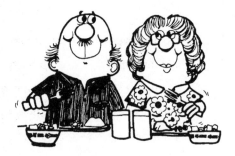

13 You Don't Have to Be Grounded

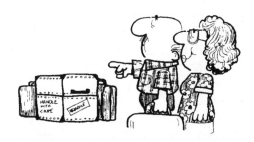

Travel is an important part of life for most people. You may need to travel for business purposes, to visit with family and friends, or just to enjoy "getting away" and seeing new places (or pleasant old ones). But when you have a breathing problem, the thought of leaving the security of home may prevent you from venturing out. Questions of safety, getting sick, and needing help may arise. For most people with chronic lung disease, however, there are relatively few contraindications to travel. With a little foresight and determination, you don't have to be grounded!

The most crucial consideration is that although you can take a vacation, there is no vacation from respiratory care. You cannot tell your lungs that you are going on a trip and will return in 2 weeks. Although your daily routine will be interrupted, you must adhere as closely as possible to your respiratory care routine. This means you must take your medications regularly and maintain hydration; if your routine includes bronchial drainage and breathing and physical training exercises, these must be continued.

The most important move you can make in planning a happy and healthful vacation is to consult your doctor, who will review your therapy and indicate whether any part of your program can be modified while you are away. Your doctor may want to give you the name of a physician at your destination whom you can contact if any difficulties arise and may even want to send a copy of your medical records ahead or with you.

In planning and preparing for your trip, you should consider some of the following travel tips:

1. When choosing your vacation site, check for the following:
   Infections. Are there any viral flu epidemics at your destination? (Of

course, you should check with your doctor about obtaining a yearly flu vaccine, regardless of known epidemics.) Does anyone you are going to visit have a cold? If so, you may want to postpone your trip.

Air pollution. How smoggy is the area? Will you have an air-conditioned room?

Allergy. If allergies play a part in your illness, avoid areas that have high pollen counts.

Altitude. Consider the altitude of the area. As we ascend, air becomes less dense and there is less oxygen available to us. At short distances above sea level this change is insignificant. But in cities at very high altitudes (that is, over 1 mile [5280 feet] high), or during air flight (the cabins are pressurized to an atmosphere equal to 1 mile high), the effect on people with chronic lung disease may be important, resulting in increased shortness of breath and other symptoms.

2. Make a checklist of your medications. Take enough to last you through the trip and for a few extra days in case of delay. It is occasionally difficult to get prescriptions from one state filled in another; nevertheless, obtain extra prescriptions from your physician as another safeguard.

3. When traveling to foreign countries, you may need a supply of general medicine (aspirin, antidiarrheal medicine, and others) with you. The quality of medications is not the same throughout the world. Avoid unknown medications, especially over-the-counter preparations, since many of these contain substances that can cause harm. Be very sure to take a sufficient supply of your prescription medications if you are going to a foreign country.

4. Establish a travel routine for your treatments, exercise, and cleaning of equipment. Write it down and follow it carefully.

5. Travel is tiring; allow time for frequent rest stops. Relax and enjoy yourself. Don't try to do too much in one day; get adequate sleep.

6. Discuss with your doctor how different altitude changes may affect you. If you need supplemental oxygen at higher altitudes, you must take it with you or arrange to have it there when you arrive.

7. If your doctor says that you will need supplemental oxygen while flying, contact the airline in advance. Most airlines won't let you bring your own equipment on board. They will supply oxygen for you for the duration of the trip. Some airlines won't allow oxygen use at all. Others require a written release from your doctor to travel and information on the amount of oxygen to be used. A few even require accompaniment by a medical person or friend. Be sure to check the rules well in advance.

8. If you use oxygen or other respiratory equipment, ask your local vendor for the name of a company that could assist you at your destination. You may have to take some of your equipment with you, but you can arrange for whatever equipment and oxygen supplies you need to be waiting for you on your arrival. (Don't forget your cleaning supplies!)

9. Go prepared for climate and weather changes. Take extra clothes for warmth and weather changes.

10. Avoid smoking areas whenever possible.

Travel makes life interesting and rewarding.
Travel whenever possible, but plan ahead.

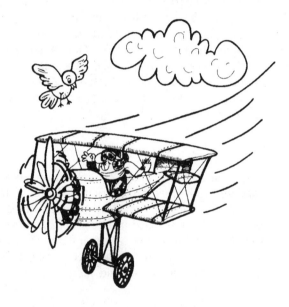

14 Smoking, Smog, and Other Bad Stuff

Avoiding irritants is a good way to prevent further damage to your lungs. People with lung disease cannot live in isolation from the rest of the world, but they can make healthful choices and educated decisions.

The causes of lung disease are complex. Our understanding of the causes of chronic lung disease and what makes it worse is far from complete. We do know that certain inhaled irritants can adversely affect your lungs. Sensible avoidance of exposure to these can help maintain your lung function and prevent deterioration.

SMOKING

Today everyone knows that cigarette smoke can impair lung function. Cigarette smoke can paralyze the hairlike projections, called cilia, in the bronchial walls. As a result, the cilia cannot move mucus toward the throat, where it is easily eliminated. Smoke also irritates the cells in the bronchial walls that produce mucus. This irritation causes inflammation, an increase in mucus production, and chronic cough. Mucus that collects in the bronchial tubes impairs the movement of air and increases the likelihood of lung infections.

People with chronic lung disease should not smoke. If you are still smoking, seek help from your local Lung Association, Heart Association, or Cancer Society. They may offer smoking cessation classes or other information available to help you. If you have tried to quit in the past, try again. Eventually you will succeed. It is important not to feel guilty or angry with yourself for having smoked in the past. Negative feelings do not help you or your lung condition.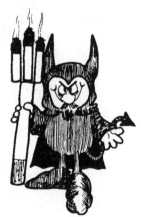

Lung cancer is another problem linked to smoking. Cancer-causing elements, known as *carcinogens*, are found in cigarette smoke. These chemical agents may cause normal cells to develop into cancerous ones. Statistically, smokers have a far greater chance of developing cancer of the lungs than do nonsmokers. Lung cancer has been a leading cause of death among American males for some years. The incidence of diagnosis of lung cancer among women has increased as the number of women who smoke has increased.

People with lung disease who continue to smoke are engaging in behavior that limits any benefit obtainable from medical treatment. The benefits derived from smoking cessation are great. You may actually *improve* your lung condition! The risk of heart disease, cancer, and the development of further lung disease may be reduced. Coughing episodes and mucus production are likely to decrease. If nothing else, you will help to preserve the lung function you have. It's worth it!

ENVIRONMENTAL EXPOSURE

Environmental factors, such as temperature and humidity, may affect your breathing. There is no "ideal" climate or environment for all patients with chronic lung disease. The environment in which you feel most comfortable is the best for you. Let's look at some environmental factors that may influence your breathing.

SECOND-HAND SMOKE

Second-hand smoke has been identified as a possible health hazard. Other people's smoke may actually harm your lungs and make you feel more short of breath. You should avoid smoke-filled places and let others know that smoke is harmful to you. Many smokers are not aware of the discomfort you may experience. Telling friends, "Yes, I do mind if you smoke" is especially difficult at first. With a little practice, it becomes easier. Here are some suggestions. Be polite and assertive when asking others not to smoke in your presence. A "No Smoking" sign on your door or desk may be sufficient. Seek out well-ventilated restaurants or "No Smoking" areas in restaurants and other public places. Avoid panic when exposed to smoke; that can be worse than any effect of smoke itself. Get involved with a local Lung Association Chapter to help educate people about the damaging effects of smoke.

AIR POLLUTION

Air pollution affects everyone, but research suggests that people with asthma, chronic bronchitis, and emphysema may have more trouble breathing when air pollution levels are high. The four major pollutants are sulfates, ozone, particles, and carbon monoxide, primarily from factories and automobile exhaust. Carbon monoxide from car exhaust interferes with the blood's ability to carry oxygen. When polluted air is exposed to the hot sun, it becomes even more irritating.

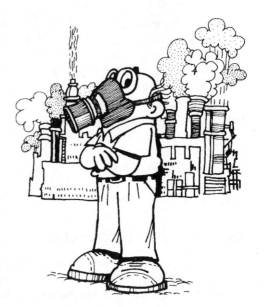

During "smog alerts," when air pollution rises to an unhealthful level, people with heart and lung disease are advised to stay indoors and avoid heavy exertion. Having air conditioning in your home may be helpful. Patients are advised to avoid rush hour traffic due to increased automobile exhaust. If you plan to travel, consider the air quality of the places you are visiting.

INDUSTRIAL POLLUTION

This occurs when the air in your workplace affects your breathing. It may be caused by dust, fumes, gases, and vapors from chemicals. Well-known industrial pollutants include asbestos and coal dust. We are discovering new forms of indoor pollution every day. Therefore, if you believe that the air in your workplace is contributing to or causing lung problems, you need to report it.

TEMPERATURE

Variations in temperature affect some people. Very cold air has been known to cause bronchospasm. Temperatures above 90° F can also affect your breathing and cause dehydration if you are not drinking enough fluids.

WET VERSUS DRY CLIMATES

The only person who can tell if a wet or dry climate is better for your breathing is you. You should visit both climates and compare.

ALLERGIES

True allergies are abnormal responses to materials that exist in the environment. For example, chopping onions makes everyone's eyes water; that is not an allergy but an irritation. It is sometimes difficult to distinguish between irritation and allergy. If you sneeze, develop a runny nose, have itchy eyes, or wheeze on exposure to certain things, you may have an allergy. It is best to avoid exposure to the allergen (substance that causes the reaction). When avoidance is not possible, allergies can be controlled with medicines such as antihistamines and corticosteroids. Discuss these possible allergies with your physician.

INFECTIONS

Infections of the lungs can be caused by viruses, fungi, or bacteria. People with lung disease often have more severe symptoms with infection because of decreased lung function. Therefore it is important to report symptoms of infection to your physician so that medical treatment can be started promptly.

Colds and influenza are caused by viruses. Annual immunization against influenza decreases the incidence of complications, hospitalization, and death due to influenza. Every year a new influenza vaccine is prepared. It provides protection against the influenza viruses expected to occur in the coming winter season. Most patients with lung disease should receive a flu shot each fall, unless otherwise advised by their physician.

A "pneumonia" vaccine is also available to protect against certain types of bacteria that cause lung infection (pneumococci). A person needs to receive this vaccine only once, not annually. It is generally recommended for patients with chronic lung disease.

Antibiotics are effective against bacteria and some fungi, but not viruses. (Drugs that affect some viruses are also now available.) But because bacterial infections may follow viral infections, patients with lung disease are often given antibiotics when they have a cold or flu.

You should talk with your doctor about when and whether you should receive these vaccines or antibiotics.

15 The Psychology of Better Breathing

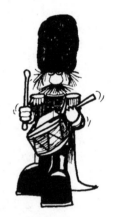

If a man does not keep pace with his companions, perhaps it is because he hears a different drummer.

H.D. Thoreau

All of us would like to be able to do what we want, when we want, and how we want. Unfortunately, we learn that many factors impose limitations. How we deal with these limitations helps determine how happy, productive, and pleasant our lives are.

Our state of health is one factor that can impose a significant limitation, and any chronic illness, such as chronic lung disease, imposes limitations permanently. A chronic limit can be particularly difficult to deal with and can make individuals angry, anxious, and depressed. Although this is understandable, it is unfortunate, because the mind and body are closely interrelated. That is, physical health can influence mental health—and vice versa. This is particularly true for people with chronic lung disease. Emotions can influence breathing in people with normal lungs; but they can have major effects on breathing when chronic lung disease is present. Therefore, dealing with your emotional or psychological self is very important to your physical health.

Saying "Deal with your emotions" or "Learn how to live with limitations" is easy; doing it is difficult. This chapter may help you by explaining the emotional problems common to persons with chronic lung disease.

In the main, there are two kinds of problems you may face: how you view yourself and how you relate to others.

YOU—THE PERSON WITH CHRONIC LUNG DISEASE

We all have a certain image of ourselves physically and emotionally. That image is critical to how we function and to how we relate to others, because our self-esteem is based on it. Chronic lung disease may be associated with a number of changes in physical image. You may gain weight because of inactivity or steroid medications, or you may lose weight because of decreased appetite. You may have noisy breathing, or you may cough and produce sputum or phlegm. You may have to walk and do other things more slowly. You may need to use oxygen in public. All of these things may impair your physical image and cause you to feel awkward, unattractive, or odd. If you feel this way, you may think that others see you the same way, and your self-esteem may suffer.

The first thing to recognize is that other people have a lot to think about besides how you look and breathe. If they do notice and ask questions, such curiosity on their part is normal. It can be satisfied by telling them the truth. You can calmly say, "It's all right, I have a lung condition and need to use oxygen"; or "It makes me cough more than I would like." Most people understand and will easily accept the truth—and you. The people who count will accept you for what you are, not how you look. People who wear casts on their legs are always asked "What happened?" A straight answer ends the curiosity, and normal interpersonal relationships can resume.

Another limitation that can bother people with chronic lung disease is their vulnerability to things over which they have no direct control. All of us are vulnerable to a number of outside forces. But with chronic lung disease, many factors may pose a special threat to well-being: infectious agents, atmospheric conditions, and environmental pollutants, for example. Such factors may lead to unpredictable changes in daily activities, which is irritating if you are used to being organized and to carefully planning your daily activities.

Chronic lung disease may lead to other alterations that can impair self-esteem. You may need to modify your work schedule or seek early retirement. You may need to modify or eliminate certain pleasurable activities such as tennis, golf, bowling, hiking, or other forms of recreation. You may need to move to seek a more favorable climate, causing you to leave behind friends and familiar surroundings. These changes can cause periods of depression, which practically all people with chronic lung disease experience.

Depression involves feelings of sadness, hopelessness, and worthlessness. The symptoms are subtle in the beginning, consisting of a lack of interest in things (possibly including your personal appearance, food, and outside activities) and fatigue. Often going out becomes a chore; friends and hobbies are abandoned. Everything becomes too much effort. Depression must be recognized early. Unless it is, the inactivity that results can worsen your condition. There is no easy antidote. You must force yourself to start moving, call friends, and go out; if necessary, seek professional help or counseling.

Certain phobias (abnormal fears of common experiences) may develop because of the real fear of becoming short of breath. For example, panic may be associated with entering closed spaces, even a shower stall. This panic worsens shortness of breath, and a terrifying vicious cycle of fear and further difficulty in breathing can result. This cycle can be prevented by learning how to control such situations with proper relaxation and breathing techniques.

Another common response to chronic lung disease (or any chronic illness) is denial. It is certainly useful to avoid becoming totally preoccupied with yourself and your illness. But denying illness can be hazardous, especially if it leads to forgetting medicines, treatments, doctor appointments, and appropriate limitations on your activity. It may lead to hiding your limitations from other people. You need to strike a balance between living within your limitations and denying their existence.

HOW YOU RELATE TO YOUR SPOUSE AND SIGNIFICANT OTHERS

Pulmonary illness has an impact not only on you, but also on your significant others, because it often alters the roles you play in relationship to others. For example, in marriage each partner usually accepts certain responsibilities. Each partner comes to rely on the other for certain activities; one may deal with finances and with social arrangements; the other may deal more effectively with certain problems or people or with house maintenance or shopping. When pulmonary illness occurs, the nature of this sharing may need to change, either temporarily or permanently. Your spouse may have to assume new roles. There is danger in this situation for both the individual with chronic lung disease and the spouse. Some people with lung disease may become more and more dependent on the healthier partner (who, in turn, may become essentially a full-time nurse). The one with chronic lung disease may fear being left alone and require more and more from the spouse, including giving up his or her outside activities and work. Both may resent the situation (often quietly)—one angry about being dependent, the other angry about becoming so depended upon. The answer is to discuss what is going on in the relationship. Excessive dependence (or doting) is to be discouraged. Both partners should do their share, even if those shares are modified in amount or nature.

Intimacy and Sexuality

To maintain an active, enjoyable sexual life, there are also certain changes that a couple may have to make when one member has lung disease. They may not be able to perform some of their previous sexual practices, since the extent of exercise tolerance may be diminished. The length of time spent in activities such as foreplay may have to be modified. In addition, certain positions previously used may no longer be comfortable and a change may be necessary. But there is no way that modifications can be made in sexual activity unless the couple is open enough to talk about sex. Also, remember that there is more to an intimate and loving relationship than just the physical activities of sex.

An unfortunate type of communication that couples frequently engage in is a game called "I hope you can read my mind." That is, one partner wishes something would change in their sexual relationship and hopes that the spouse will comply with the unspoken wish. The ice may have to be broken by one person who just comes out and talks about it. As an example, one woman was required to use oxygen for any type of exertion, including sexual activity. She felt that having her oxygen tank in the bedroom detracted from the sexual atmosphere during relations with her husband. Her solution was to place the tank outside the bedroom and use a long tube that reached the bed. There is no reason for sexual activity to stop because a person has lung disease. The key is to be open about it, and then modify the activity to that which is physically possible.

Friends

If you have a negative image of yourself, it may interfere with your friendships. You may begin to fear that you are more trouble than you are worth— that you are a burden to others. Your response may be to withdraw from relationships or to try and maintain a facade (doing more than you should really do). Again, the fact is that your friends rarely share these same feelings (that you are a burden) and will respect and understand your limits. If you ask them to walk more slowly, to not smoke around you, or to alter social plans, almost all will understand and respond. But you can't play "read my mind." You must tell your friends about your limits rather than try to hide them. You can take an active role in planning your social life so that it fits within your limitations. There is no need to be totally left out.

THE BOTTOM LINE

We have reviewed some of the common problems faced by patients with lung disease and some of the feelings they may develop. There are some very important principles you must remember to help you maintain both a positive state of mental health and a good quality of life. First, having a lung disease does not necessarily mean you must give up certain activities in your life. Instead, you should modify your activities and still be involved in them. Many people have difficulty learning to pace themselves, but with patience and practice, it can be done. For example, people who are distraught that they can no longer play 18 holes of golf may find that it is possible to play 9 holes with a cart. Patient and spouse can enjoy golf again—a pleasure they thought was gone forever. When you have lung disease, you may develop misconceptions as to the safe limits of physical exertion; that is, once you begin to develop shortness of breath, you may stop the activity instead of slowing it down. There is a tendency to stop sooner and sooner in the activity, and consequently, to begin to feel that you can do very little. Although you may have to slow down, you can learn that if you push yourself a little, you can do more than you thought. Doing more will improve your self-esteem and endurance. The important thing is to figure out how you can do what you like. Don't give it up! Rearrange it! Adapt it to your needs! Soon the new pace will no longer be planned; it will become natural to you. You can continue to be involved with your family, with your friends, and with the world.

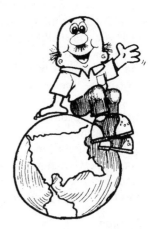

Another important principle is to learn as much as possible about your illness. You should try to learn about your lung function, your medicines, and your treatments. Ask questions of doctors, nurses, and therapists, as well as other people with chronic lung disease until you have obtained answers. The process of educating yourself about your illness has enormous psychological value. As you know more about your illness, some of the unfounded fears can be dispelled. In addition, as you develop more understanding, you can play a more active role in keeping yourself healthy and helping yourself when you are ill. A great deal can be learned not only from medical personnel, but also from others with lung disease. People with chronic lung disease have accumulated a vast amount of experience about how to live successfully within the physical limits that exist. You can share their experiences, contribute your own, and give each other support. This can be done through rehabilitation programs, at American Lung Association meetings, and in informal groups.

The essence of good psychological health is to maintain a positive attitude toward living, while still knowing the facts and being realistic. Remain as active as possible, and try to maintain your sense of humor. Your life is not "over" because of lung disease; it is changed, but you can enjoy this changed life greatly if you maintain a positive image of yourself. Remember always to focus on what you *can* do, not just on what you *can't*.

16 When to Call Your Doctor and What to Do in an Emergency

Most people with *chronic lung disease* have regularly scheduled visits with their doctor. But when should you call your doctor between these visits? Usually, in discussions with your doctor, details are worked out to cover this question. In general, however, there are two major "signals" that your doctor will want to know about:

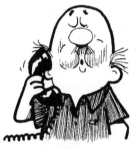

1. Any *change* in your symptoms, particularly if this change lasts more than 1 day

2. Any *new symptoms* that you develop

Obviously, we all have our ups and downs, our good days and bad. But changes and new symptoms should be called to your doctor's attention.

Some of the *changes* or *new symptoms* that might be important are:

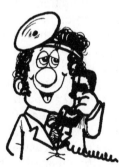

- Fever
- Increased shortness of breath, added difficulty in breathing, or increased wheezing (more than usual)
- Increased coughing (more frequent, more severe, or both)
- Increased sputum production
- Change in color of sputum (to yellow, gray, or green)
- Change in consistency of sputum (thicker)
- Swelling of ankles, legs, or around eyes
- Sudden weight gain (3 to 5 pounds overnight)
- Palpitations of the heart or pulse faster than usual
- Unusual dizziness, sleepiness, headaches, visual disturbances, irritability, or trouble thinking
- Loss of appetite (more than usual)
- Dehydration (evidenced by concentrated urine and dryness of skin)
- Chest pains
- Blood in sputum, urine, or bowel movement

You should discuss these "signals" with your doctor, who may want you to change your medicines or add new ones (for example, to increase fluid intake and/or to start a preselected antibiotic for fever and increased cough). The more thoroughly you work out these signals ahead of time, the better you will be able to deal with these changes, and the less frequently you will have to call your doctor on an emergency basis. But when in doubt, check it out with your doctor.

WHAT TO DO IN AN EMERGENCY

Many patients and their spouses and/or family members want to know what to do in an emergency. There are three things that will make it rather simple to deal with this question:

1. Become familiar with what an "emergency" is
2. Know what options for medical care are open to you
3. Have a *plan*

In general, an "emergency" is some *sudden change* or *new development* in your condition, particularly changes or new things that impair your ability to function or that frighten you. Sudden and/or severe chest pains or shortness of breath are the most common "emergencies" in patients with chronic lung diseases. Coughing up blood is another. So *sudden changes* in your condition and *new symptoms* of a major kind usually constitute a true emergency.

Of course, many patients with lung disease have mild changes that are frightening and may cause panic. Other sections of this book offer methods for dealing with panic. For example, if breathing becomes more difficult, you should assume a sitting position and lean forward slightly; pursed lip breathing usually helps, as may using relaxation techniques (see Chapter 10). Inhalation of a bronchodilator aerosol (see Chapter 5) is useful if the shortness of breath is caused by bronchospasm. You must learn how to deal with such episodes; discussions with your doctor about these and other maneuvers will help.

But what if the symptoms are severe, don't go away, or are new? This constitutes a true emergency. In this situation, most patients want to see their doctor *immediately*, and that is a good idea because he or she knows you best. But that may not be possible or even in your best interest in an emergency. The key to making an emergency plan is, again, a discussion with your doctor. You should determine when he/she is available (no one is available 24 hours a day, 7 days a week!); how you can contact him/her; and, if your doctor is not available when you try to contact him/her, what you should do. Many doctors have associates who "take calls" when they themselves are not available; some do not. If you cannot contact your own physician (or associates), what should you do—call an ambulance or the

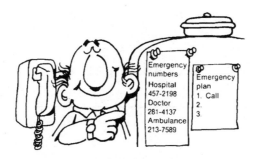

paramedics? If you do that, to what emergency facility should you be taken?

The answer to these questions will be different in different communities. In general, an "emergency" means you need prompt access to medical care. Obviously, it is an advantage if your doctor (or associate) is available to provide your medical history, even if he/she cannot be physically present.

Therefore, the important thing is to *plan ahead* so you know what to do. Have a written "plan" near the telephone: *names* of *whom to call* and the *proper telephone numbers*: your primary doctor, "backup" doctors, ambulance or paramedic numbers, and location of the nearest emergency facility. Think through the situation ahead of time; put yourself in the place of your spouse or friend, as if you were helping *him/her* in an emergency. Once you have a plan, there is no reason for anyone to panic in an emergency. So worry about it *now* and get it worked out *now*. Hopefully, you will never need to put it into action!

Many patients don't want to "bother" their doctor; but whether your symptoms warrant "bothering" your doctor should be decided by the doctor. As you get to know each other and you become more knowledgeable, this decision will become easier. Err on the side of "bothering" whenever you are uncertain.

Getting It All Together

Now that you have been introduced to various self-care techniques, schedule your activities and therapies into a workable daily plan. Completing a daily schedule can help you develop a workable, balanced regimen of treatments, rest, exercise, and recreation. Start by listing what you need to do each day. Include all the key elements of your particular program: medications, bronchial drainage, 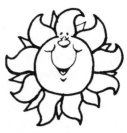 breathing exercises, aerosol treatments, arm exercises, walks, and special meals.

It is important to set a realistic schedule to ensure a positive, successful outcome. You will have to push yourself at times as you work toward improving your strength and endurance, but the rewards will be worth the effort.

The sequence of your program is important. Here are some tips:

- Bronchial drainage needs to be done before meals or no sooner than 1 hour after meals.
- Inhaled bronchodilator and mist-producing machines (nebulizers, etc.) should be used before bronchial drainage and generally before exercise.
- Plan to walk at your best time of the day. Do not exercise or walk immediately after a meal. Wait at least an hour; or do your exercises before eating.
- Remember to schedule naps, rest periods, snacks, and fluids throughout the day.

An example of a typical daily schedule is on the following page. With the help of your doctor, nurse, or therapist, fill in the blank schedule, using the example as a guide.

SAMPLE SCHEDULE

Morning

1. After awakening, take bronchodilator medication (pill), if prescribed.

2. Take inhaled bronchodilator, if prescribed.

3. Perform bronchial drainage within 30 minutes of taking inhaled bronchodilator.

4. Eat breakfast.

5. After at least an hour, walk at designated speed and for prescribed time. (Practice breathing exercises while walking.)

6. Have a nutritious snack with a glass of water.

7. Rest.

8. Have more liquids (space fluid intake throughout day and keep a careful record of amounts).

9. After you feel rested, do arm exercises and/or stretching exercises.

Afternoon

1. Eat lunch.

2. Take medications, if prescribed.

3. After at least an hour, practice breathing exercises and relaxation techniques in a quiet setting.

4. If you are walking more than once a day, walk again at your designated speed and time. (Remember breathing exercises while walking.)

5. Have a snack with a glass of water.

6. Do arm exercises and/or stretching exercises.

7. Drink more liquids.

Evening

1. Eat dinner.

2. If you are walking more than twice a day, take another walk at your designated speed and for the appropriate time.

3. Do arm exercises.

4. Take medications.

5. An hour or more before bedtime, use bronchodilator aerosol.

6. Perform bronchial drainage within 30 minutes.

7. Clean nebulizer equipment (if applicable).

8. Perform relaxation techniques.

MODIFYING YOUR SCHEDULE

If you work outside the home, you can adapt your daily program of care. For example:

1. You may need to get up earlier to allow plenty of time to do bronchial drainage. You will feel more like "tackling" the day if your lungs are clear of mucus.

2. If bronchial drainage is not part of your program, you might choose to take your walk before getting ready for work.

3. Arrange to take a short walk at lunch time, then eat your lunch afterward.

4. A good way to remind yourself to drink fluids throughout the day is to have a pitcher or thermos of water, juice, or other beverage readily available on your desk or nearby.

5. At break time, find a quiet place where you can relax. Practice relaxation techniques or breathing exercises at this time.

6. Do breathing techniques periodically throughout the day while working.

Do not forget time for *activities you enjoy*. Arrange your schedule so that it includes time for some of your favorite hobbies and activities. These are important for your mental health!

YOUR DAILY SCHEDULE

Morning

1. _____

2. _____

3. _____

4. _____

5. _____

6. _____

Afternoon

1. _____

2. _____

3. _____

4. _____

5. _____

6. _____

Evening

1. _____

2. _____

3. _____

4. _____

5. _____

6. _____

18 You Don't Have to Do It Alone: Pulmonary Rehabilitation

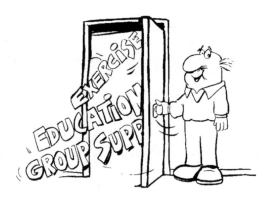

So far in this book we have discussed some general and specific health care measures that are important for the person with chronic lung disease. Learning more about chronic lung disease and your own condition is an important step in improving your quality of life. In many areas, pulmonary rehabilitation programs run by health professionals who are experienced in helping patients with lung diseases have been established. Their goal: to help patients learn more about their disease and to cope better with it.

Rehabilitation is defined as "the restoration of the individual to the fullest medical, mental, emotional, social, and vocational potential of which he/she is capable." A *pulmonary* rehabilitation program is one which specializes in the rehabilitation of individuals with chronic lung disease.

People with chronic lung disease, like all individuals, can live fuller and more productive lives if they *actively* participate in their own health care and have the *tools* with which to do so. Pulmonary rehabilitation is a preventive health care program provided by a team of health care professionals, a program designed to help you acquire these tools. The primary goals of a pulmonary rehabilitation program are to provide you with the proper information, education, specific self-care therapies, and support to help stabilize your illness and improve your quality of life. Specific aims of pulmonary rehabilitation are as follows:

1. To teach patients, their family members, and their significant others about chronic lung disease, its effects and consequences, and ways to minimize or control the problems that chronic lung disease may cause.

2. To maximize physical strength and exercise tolerance.

3. To reduce your symptoms and help you gain control over them.

4. To enhance emotional well-being.

5. To help you cope with the limitations and frustrations caused by having chronic lung disease.

6. To increase self-confidence and independence.

7. To help you become a more *active* partner in your relationship with your physician.

WHAT ARE THE COMPONENTS OF A PULMONARY REHABILITATION PROGRAM?

Evaluation

Like any other person with chronic lung disease, you can be considered for participation in a pulmonary rehabilitation program if you are *motivated* to learn more about your condition and to help yourself. An interview with a team member is an important part of the assessment process. During the interview, the program is explained, any questions are answered, and medical records are reviewed. A specific program can then be designed to meet *your* individual needs.

Physical Therapy

Good bronchial hygiene, effective coughing, clapping, and bronchial drainage may be taught as part of a self-care program. Instruction in diaphragmatic breathing exercises and pursed lip breathing is stressed and reinforced. These measures are designed to reduce the work of breathing and to increase your ability to perform daily activities.

Respiratory Therapy Equipment

Instruction may be provided in the proper use and cleaning of respiratory therapy equipment (e.g., metered dose inhaler, spacer, extender, or nebulizer). Your potential need for supplemental oxygen can be evaluated. If any equipment is needed, instruction will be provided regarding its proper use.

Education

Active patient participation is important. Therefore, you and your family members should *understand* your underlying disease process as well as the kinds of activity you can perform safely. Team members will discuss with you topics such as the purpose of your medications and their side effects, proper nutrition, identifying signs and symptoms of a respiratory tract infection, and self-care tips. They will also help you to plan a daily schedule.

Exercise

A physical conditioning program is an important component of pulmonary rehabilitation, since it has been shown to improve exercise capacity for individuals with chronic lung disease. After a thorough initial evaluation, the team will select an appropriate and safe exercise routine tailored to your needs, supervise you during the initial stages, and prescribe a safe routine for you to follow at home.

Feelings and Emotions

Successful rehabilitation requires attention not only to *physical* problems but also to *psychological, emotional,* and *social* ones. Understandably, individuals with chronic illness often have difficulty dealing with the limitations and symptoms caused by their illness. One symptom in particular, *shortness of breath,* is closely linked to your emotional state. The sensation of shortness of breath may lead to anxiety and fear, which may then cause more shortness of breath and discomfort; this may lead you into a vicious cycle. Support groups may help you to feel less isolated and alone. These groups also provide a forum in which you can share feelings, frustrations, hopes, and joys.

Benefits of Pulmonary Rehabilitation

Through the years, research has shown that there are measurable benefits from participating in a comprehensive pulmonary rehabilitation program. Some of these benefits follow:

1. Increased knowledge about lung disease.
2. Increased exercise capacity.
3. Improved ability to perform activities of daily living.
4. Decreased sensation of shortness of breath.
5. Decreased anxiety and panic.
6. Improved quality of life.
7. Decreased time spent in hospitals.

These benefits are certainly encouraging, but it must be stressed that it takes a motivated, committed person to participate in pulmonary rehabilitation and make the necessary changes to improve his/her life. With a little help from a team of qualified, supportive, and caring health professionals, these benefits may be within your reach.

WHERE ARE PULMONARY REHABILITATION PROGRAMS LOCATED?

Pulmonary rehabilitation programs exist nationwide. Ask your physician, friends, a local hospital, or the American Lung Association for information on a nearby program. Also, the American Association of Cardiovascular and Pulmonary Rehabilitation publishes a nationwide directory.

If *you* are ready, there are programs ready for you!

19 A Look to the Future

Medical research is constantly working toward the answers to many of the mysteries about lung diseases.

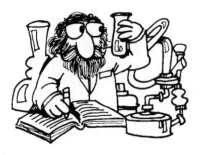

In cases of COPD, research on emphysema has indicated that the destruction of elastic tissue in the air sacs probably results from digestion of this tissue by an enzyme called *elastase*. This enzyme is normally carried around the body in white blood cells. We also know that a blood protein called alpha-1-antitrypsin (also called alpha-1-proteinase inhibitor or alpha-1-Pi or just a-1-Pi) can *inhibit* (prevent or block) the effects of elastase. Some persons have an inherited deficiency of alpha-1-Pi and get emphysema early in life, but this deficiency is rare. A-1-Pi has been purified and is now available to give to individuals born with this deficiency. Why the elastase-inhibitor system becomes unbalanced in patients who do not have a *hereditary* a-1-Pi deficiency is not clear. It is known that oxidants, including those in cigarette smoke, can render a-1-Pi *inactive*. Intensive research is focused on whether this inactivation, and other factors, lead to lung injury. If we learn this, we should be able to develop drugs to prevent this injury. Indeed, new drugs that block elastase and oxidants are under development.

The causes of chronic bronchitis also are being studied. Clearly, there is an association with cigarette smoking and certain industrial exposures— but why? What inhalants are responsible? What makes the bronchial tubes behave the way they do? Can we develop drugs that will thin mucus effectively or prevent excess mucus production or stop the inflammation of the bronchial tube lining? We probably can and will.

Existing drugs and treatments for COPD are constantly being refined, and new ones are being developed. Just within the last few years, several new medicines have been introduced that relieve spasm of bronchial tubes or relieve inflammation of the mucous membranes. These are better than our older medicines in that they may either have fewer side effects or longer duration of action, are in a more convenient form to take, may prevent spasm (rather than treat it after it occurs), or may be more effective or less costly. Although "new" does not necessarily mean "better," some of these "new" medicines may be "better" for you.

Another example of what lies ahead concerns drugs for better treatment of infection. As discussed earlier, infections are caused by different kinds of invaders—bacteria, fungi, and viruses. Antibiotics are effective in treating infections caused by bacteria. Unfortunately, they are not that effective against fungi and are not useful at all against viruses. No antibiotic can treat the flu and other viral infections. But research already has provided some drugs that can prevent (or treat) certain kinds of viral and fungal infections, and the future in this area looks bright.

Lung transplantation is another area of intense interest. Questions that need answers include the following: Who *needs* a lung transplant? W*hen* should it be done? Is one "new" lung enough (versus two)? How can we preserve a potential donor lung longer (now it must be used within 3 to 6 hours after removal)? How can we prevent lung rejection? There are many more questions than answers right now. However, a number of patients with severe chronic lung disease have already received lung transplants, and the pace is accelerating.

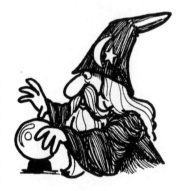

Despite the many questions that remain, we clearly have made substantial gains. Some of the biggest gains have been in *education of the public* about the factors that contribute to disease. Young children are being taught the hazards of smoking in the hope that they will never *begin* to smoke. Smokers are being aided in their efforts to quit. Many agencies are working toward cleaning up our air, another source of lung pollution.

We are becoming aware of certain hazards in the *workplace* (with asbestos being the most publicized) and are making progress in decreasing such hazards. Everywhere in our country, doctors and other medical personnel are becoming increasingly aware of chronic lung disease and are being trained in modern diagnosis and management.

The more that medical research discovers about chronic lung disease, the better doctors will be able to treat their patients. The *ultimate* goal is to learn enough so that chronic lung disease can be prevented. The key to achieving that goal is to ensure that skilled researchers are trained and provided with the tools they need to continue the present pace of advancement.

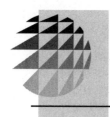

Index